AUTOPSY PATHOLOGY
PROCEDURE AND PROTOCOL

AUTOPSY PATHOLOGY PROCEDURE AND PROTOCOL

By

DUDLEY L. WEBER, M.D.

EUGENE P. FAZZINI, M.D.

THOMAS J. REAGAN, M.D.

Department of Pathology
New York University Medical Center
Bellevue Hospital
New York, New York

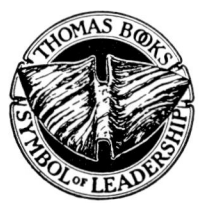

CHARLES C THOMAS • PUBLISHER
Springfield • Illinois • U.S.A.

Published and Distributed Throughout the World by
CHARLES C THOMAS • PUBLISHER
BANNERSTONE HOUSE
301-327 East Lawrence Avenue, Springfield, Illinois, U.S.A.

This book is protected by copyright. No
part of it may be reproduced in any manner
without written permission from the publisher.

© *1973, by* CHARLES C THOMAS • PUBLISHER
ISBN 0-398-02625-4
Library of Congress Catalog Card Number: 72-81722

With THOMAS BOOKS *careful attention is given to all details of manufacturing and design. It is the Publisher's desire to present books that are satisfactory as to their physical qualities and artistic possibilities and appropriate for their particular use.* THOMAS BOOKS *will be true to those laws of quality that assure a good name and good will.*

Printed in the United States of America
Q-1

*to the residents of Bellevue Hospital
past, present, future*

PREFACE

It is the purpose of this book to present the fundamentals of autopsy technique. Methods for the description and recording of harvested observations are described. In most cases, alternate methods for the performance of a given procedure are presented.

The authors do not intend this work as a text of differential diagnosis in autopsy pathology. We hope to present methods which have been found to be valuable in the performance of autopsies and to instruct the young pathologist in his first attempts at organizing his procedure.

It is our hope that the reader, as he gains in experience, will proceed to modify these techniques to his own use in accordance with his needs and practices.

The two principal methods of autopsy, namely those of Virchow and Rokitansky, will be discussed and outlined in detail. Alternate methods of protocol will be shown in the hope that the one best suited to the prosectors' needs might be adopted. A section on accident investigation is included, since in many areas which do not have a trained forensic pathologist available, this task falls to the general hospital pathologist. It is the opinion of the authors that general pathologists not familiar with forensic pathology defer such investigations (as homicide and suicide) to an expert in the field, even at the cost of summoning one from the nearest available point.

Dudley L. Weber
Eugene P. Fazzini
Thomas J. Reagan

INTRODUCTION AND HISTORICAL CONSIDERATIONS

No method of inquiry may be said to be scientific if observation and control of results are not possible. The beginning of scientific medicine may then be assumed to be the point at which autopsy, which allowed investigation into the accuracy of diagnosis and efficiency of therapy, became a reality.

Early records are blurred; however, it appears that autopsies were performed at the Medical School of the University of Bologna in the early fourteenth century. A record kept in the Archives of that University reveals that an autopsy was performed in a case of suspected poisoning. It is apparent from the protocol that the investigation was ordered by the court. The earliest application of autopsy technique was therefore for forensic purposes. It fell to Antonio Benivieni, a Florentine physician, to request permission from the family of deceased patients to be allowed to perform autopsies in cases of death which were of apparently natural causes. The autopsy now had as its purpose the investigation of these causes as they are revealed in structural alterations.

Riva in the mid-seventeenth century established a museum of pathological anatomy in Rome. Riva also founded the first known pathological society.

Morgagni produced the first text in the field of pathological anatomy, *Seats and Causes of Disease*. In this work several hundred of the masters' autopsies were collected. Among the French, such names as Laennec and Corvisart are of prominence as early founders of the science of pathology.

Hunter, Bright, Addison and Hodgkin of Guys Hospital are but a few of the brilliant British contributors. In America the earliest known text was written by Dr. Samuel D. Gross of Jefferson Medical College in Philadelphia.

The grandeur of Austro-Germanic pathology is often lost to the present generation. Consideration of the former greatness of these centers is obfuscated by clear-cut recent memories of the inhuman horrors perpetrated against humanity by some of the latter-day practitioners trained in these once great schools. Certainly the names of Virchow and Rokitansky must be dissocated from those of some of their latter-day descendents.

Rudolph Virchow can clearly be considered the father of modern pathology. The concept put forth in his text, *Die Allgemeine Celluläre Pathology*, namely that disease is produced by a reaction between the offending agent and the host tissues, led to the application of microscopy as an essential part of anatomic pathology. Virchow's method of dissection, to be described in a later section, is one of the two principal methods of dissection.

The method of Rokitansky, also to be described in a later section, was popularized by his student Hanns Chiari in a book published in the late nineteenth century.

Modern pathology has been implemented by histochemistry tissue culture and electron microscopy. In recent years the drama of the modern mechanized clinical laboratory has captured the fascination of many pathologists. The autopsy room remains, however, the point where the final significance of these chemically derived parameters may be evaluated in terms of health and disease.

For reasons which are not clear to the authors, forensic and hospital pathology have in many areas been dissociated to the point where, save for some large metropolitan centers, forensic pathology has been relegated to a coroner's system. In some areas where a medical examiner's system exists, the medical examiner is not a pathologist or has only the most rudimentary acquaintance with pathology. The tragedy lies in the fact that forensic questions of the greatest consequence are often left to be decided by inexperienced and poorly trained practitioners.

Among the great contributors to American forensic pathology are: Dr. Charles Norris, first Chief Medical Examiner of the City of New York; Dr. Milton Helpern, present Chief Medical Examiner of that city; Dr. Alan Moritz of Ohio; and Dr. Russell Fisher of Maryland, all of whom are among the great pathologists and teachers of pathology on the American scene.

Neuropathology has often also shared the sad fate of forensic pathology. The study of the central nervous system has in many places been relegated to nonpathologists, often neurologists, who, expert as they may be in their own fields, have little if any formal training in general pathology upon which to base their anatomic investigations of the nervous system. This condition has in recent years been greatly improved through the efforts of such teachers as Dr. Abner Wolf, Dr. Irwin Feigin, and Dr. Kenneth Earle, all of whom base their sound understanding of neuropathology on fundamentals of general morbid anatomy.

It is apparent from the above that the authors consider autopsy pathology to be the fundamental training ground both for the pathologist and for the clinician. The autopsy room is indeed the reference point for all medical practice.

The authors of this book gratefully
acknowledge the assistance of
Miss Rosalyn Klein, Miss Gail Ciccio,
the typists for the book, and
Mr. Robert Waldeck, the photographer.

CONTENTS

	Page
Preface	vii
Introduction and Historical Considerations	ix

Chapter

1.	GENERAL CONSIDERATIONS	3
2.	AUTOPSY METHODS AND PROCEDURES	10
3.	THE NERVOUS SYSTEM	40
4.	SPECIAL PROCEDURES	67
5.	ACCIDENT PATHOLOGY	71
6.	AUTOPSY INFORMATION	75

Appendix—Organ Weights	115
Index	117

AUTOPSY PATHOLOGY
PROCEDURE AND PROTOCOL

Chapter 1

GENERAL CONSIDERATIONS

PERMISSION FOR AUTOPSY

It is necessary to obtain consent for an autopsy from the proper source. In some jurisdictions failure to do so with subsequent performance of an autopsy constitutes assault on the body of the decedent and may be interpreted as a felony or aggravated misdemeanor. Consent should be sought from the nearest relation.

In New York the following sequence of relationship obtains:

- surviving spouse
- surviving children
- parents
- siblings
- children of siblings
- grandparents
- aunts and uncles
- cousins

When more than one person of the proper degree of kinship exists, it is best to obtain written permission from all. The written consent of a single person of this group is acceptable if no objection has been raised by any other member of this group.

When there are no known surviving relatives the law varies from one jurisdiction to another. In some areas a friend who will assume responsibility for burial of the body may give consent for autopsy immediately. In other areas, although the consent be given, the autopsy may not be performed for a given period of time, usually 48 hours, permitting a search for relatives.

When a body is unclaimed by a relative or friend, many states have provisions for disposition of the body to medical schools or other institutions. In New York a certain percentage of unclaimed bodies (in New York City 20%) are released for autopsy on order of the director of mortuaries when requested by the clinical service or physician attending the patient. In all cases the local laws must be consulted prior to performing an autopsy.

None of the restrictions noted apply in cases when an autopsy is ordered by a medical examiner or coroner in a case of death of suspicious origin. This is discussed in greater detail in the chapter devoted to medicolegal autopsies and medical examiners' cases. In general, these cases include suspected homicide, suicide, deaths following trauma or related to drug abuse including alcoholism and patients dying unexpectedly while not under the care of a physician. When a case falls into the category of a medical examiners' case, it is imperative that consent not be sought before the case is reported to the medical examiner to avoid the difficulties encountered when consent is denied and the medical examiner subsequently orders an autopsy.

Autopsies on military personnel may be ordered at the discretion of the commander of the military post. If the death occurs in any way that would ordinarily place it in the category of a medical examiner's case, it is usually subject to the jurisdiction of the local medical examiner within the United States. Again it is necessary to consult local laws (and treaty agreements with foreign countries) before proceeding with an autopsy.

The consent form must include the patients' name, unit number, the name of the person(s)

S.R. 1485 (Rev. '63)–10M-427158(66) 114

....Hospital

**THE CITY OF NEW YORK
DEPARTMENT OF HOSPITALS**

AUTHORIZATION FOR AUTOPSY

Date..

I (We) ...., the..and next of kin of..who died on..19.........., grant the ....Hospital permission to perform an autopsy on the body of said deceased for the purpose of determining the cause of death and studying any disease processes found; the extent of the autopsy to be as follows:

....

I (We) further authorize the retention of such parts and tissues as the pathologist may consider necessary for the foregoing purposes:

Signature(s) and Address(es) of Witness(es):   Signature(s) and Address(es) of Next of Kin:

The undersigned does hereby authorize..Hospital (subject only to such restrictions, if any, as may set forth below) to remove either or both eyes from the body of said deceased and to retain and use either or both eyes for such purposes as the members of the Hospital Staff or the members of the Staff of the Eye Bank for Sight Restoration, Inc., in their discretion may think necessary or desirable.

Restrictions, if any :..

....

Signature(s) and Address(es) of Witness(es):   Signature(s) and Address(es) of Next of Kin:

Approved..Hospital Administrator

....Pathologist

Figure 1. An autopsy permit.

giving consent with the degree of relationship and address(es). The extent of the autopsy must be stated with any restrictions. In some states "no restrictions" is acceptable. In others it must be clearly stated "complete including thorax, abdomen and head." It is especially important to include permission for special examinations such as eyes or extremities. The consent must also include permission for retention of tissue deemed by the pathologist to be necessary for diagnosis. The consent may also include a space for a statement of the time that the remains will be released. There should be a space for the signature of a witness to the consent. Many hospitals require that a hospital administrator approve the consent before the case is delivered to the pathologist.

A sample form as used in the New York City Municipal Hospitals is illustrated (Fig. 1).

Although it is always best to obtain written consent, many jurisdictions permit telegram consents, and some permit telephoned consents if the call is witnessed by an operator.

Common-law Spouse Consent

In many states so-called common-law marriages are legally recognized as valid marriages usually after cohabitation of a designated number of years. In some states the common-law spouse is legally recognized as the next of kin for purposes of autopsy consent. In other states common-law marriages may be recognized but not for purposes of autopsy consent when the common-law spouse may have only the status of "friend," willing or unwilling to assume burial expenses. The status as common-law spouses must be determined according to local jurisdiction before proceeding with attempts to secure autopsy permission.

In all cases the local laws must be consulted prior to performing an autopsy.

RELIGIOUS CONSIDERATIONS

In large metropolitan centers of the United States various ethnic, racial, and religious groups are to be found. Each has its own usage and belief. Some groups have no objection to autopsy. Other groups most strongly oppose it.

It is not our purpose to argue the various beliefs but to present a brief summary of them and where possible their rationale, so that the practicing pathologist might understand the various objections to autopsy which he might encounter in his practice.

Roman Catholics have no religious objection to autopsy. Most Protestant denominations do not offer objections to autopsy although some fundamentalist groups do.

The three major Jewish denominations in the United States are not unified in their teachings regarding autopsy. Reformed Judaism is not opposed to the performance of autopsy. All Orthodox and most Conservative congregations do oppose autopsy. We learn from the *Encyclopedia of the Jewish Religion* (Holt, Rinehart, and Winston) that autopsy is not allowed in the Orthodox congregations because of the biblical injunction in Deuteronomy 21:23 to enter the body in every part without delay immediately after death.

Those Protestant groups objecting to autopsy also do so based on the above stated grounds.

DEATH CERTIFICATE

A properly completed death certificate is mandated in all jurisdictions. The death certificate serves the dual purpose of registering the cause of death and optimally providing statistical data as to the prevalence of various diseases in the community. Many medical reports and correlations depend on accurate reporting on death certificates, and clearly those based on adequate postmortem examination will be the most accurate. The death certificate used in New York is illustrated (Fig. 2). It follows an internationally recommended format. The immediate cause of death with duration is listed first, followed by antecedent conditions (with duration) leading to the immediate cause of death. Other pathologic lesions are listed separately.

It is highly desirable that the death certificate be signed after completion of the autopsy. If performance of the postmortem examination is delayed because of absence of next of kin or delay in finding the nearest of kin, the physician who treated the patient will usually be required to submit the death certificate within 24 hours. In such cases the pathologist may submit an amended certificate if his findings differ significantly from those of the attending physician. This is most important when evidence of

Figure 2. Death certificate used in New York City.

17H (Rev. 68)

Certificate No...

PHYSICIAN'S CONFIDENTIAL MEDICAL REPORT

I am submitting herewith a confidential report of the cause of death of:

N.B. Enter only one cause each for (a), (b), and (c).

FULL NAME OF DECEASED (Type or Print)	22. COLOR OR RACE OF DECEDENT
John Arthur Doe	Caucasian

23. DEATH WAS CAUSED BY: (Describe Below)

			INTERVAL BETWEEN ONSET AND DEATH
(1) a. IMMEDIATE CAUSE. This does not mean the mode of dying such as heart failure, asthenia, etc. It means the disease or complication which caused death.	PART 1	a. Immediate Cause: Acute pulmonary edema	3 hours
b. and c. ANTECEDENT CAUSES. Morbid conditions, if any, giving rise to the above cause (a) stating the underlying cause last.		b. Due to or as a consequence of: Infarct of myocardium (left ventricle)	6 days
		c. Due to or as a consequence of: Atherosclerosis of coronary arteries	years
2 Conditions contributing to the death, but not related to the terminal condition mentioned in Part 1. (a)	PART 2	Other Significant Conditions: Carcinoma of kidney, left	unknown

24. IF DEATH OF FEMALE
- Any history of pregnancy in last 6 months? N/A
- If so, was she delivered? N/A
- If Yes, date of delivery: N/A
- Liveborn or stillborn? N/A

25. OPERATION
- Date of (If none, so state): None
- Major findings of operation: N/A

26. AUTOPSY—Date of (If none, so state): 17 December 1972

Signature: Richard Roe ~~D.O.~~ M.D. Address: Bellevue Hospital

BUREAU OF RECORDS AND STATISTICS—DEPARTMENT OF HEALTH—THE CITY OF NEW YORK

Figure 3. Physician's confidential medical report.

medicolegal significance is discovered. If there is a medical examiner system in your county, the medical examiner will be required to sign the death certificate, and the pathologist must never sign it unless deputized to do so by the medical examiner.

If after completion of the study of all organs there are microscopically additional significant diseases not apparent on gross examination, these findings should be reported to the local health authorities even if the disease did not directly contribute to the patient's death. For example, should a patient die of myocardial infarction but also have a microscopic area of bronchogenic carcinoma, that fact should be added to the death certificate for statistical purposes.

JURISDICTION OF MEDICAL EXAMINER

The laws regulating the jurisdiction of the medical examiner vary from city to city. It is impossible to present in this work the various laws which prevail in the United States. We have therefore chosen to present the laws determining medical examiners jurisdiction in the City of New York. Cases are placed in two major groups.

Group I

Cases with impelling legal implications in which an autopsy is usually performed by the medical examiner and in which permission for autopsy should never be requested by the hospital physician:

1. Deaths by homicide.

2. Deaths by suicide or suspicion of suicide.
3. Deaths due to injury.
4. Deaths resulting from abortion.
5. Deaths from poisoning including bacterial poisoning.

Group II

Deaths where the medical examiner may decide that it is not necessary for him to do an autopsy as part of his postmortem investigation.

1. Deaths during or immediately following diagnostic or therapeutic surgical or anaesthetic procedure.
2. Deaths occurring in an unusual or peculiar manner, or when the patient was unattended by a physician or following coma, or convulsive seizure, the cause of which is not evident.
3. Deaths resulting from chronic alcoholism.
4. Deaths in which traumatic injury was contributory and did not arise out of negligence or arson or assault.

When in the performance of an autopsy a pathologist discovers evidence of injury or disease which might place the case in the jurisdiction of the medical examiners, such as finding an unsuspected acute subdural hematoma, it is his duty to stop the autopsy and inform the medical examiner by telephone. He will then be instructed by the medical examiner as to whether he is to proceed or have the body transferred to the medical examiner's office. In Group II cases the medical examiner might instruct the hospital pathologist to proceed with the case if he has consent and will then review the gross findings. If death is then seen by the medical examiner to be due to natural causes, he may either relinquish jurisdiction and allow the hospital pathologist to issue the death certificate or retain jurisdiction and issue the certificate himself. Obviously where doubt exists by the hospital the medical examiner should be consulted.

THE PATHOLOGIST AND THE FUNERAL DIRECTOR

To paraphrase a song title of the 1940's, "the pathologist and the funeral director should be friends." If the pathologist can establish a good working relationship with the local funeral directors there will be no charges of "mutilation of the body," "butchering," etc. that sometimes occur.

The establishment of that rapport is easier in small communities than in large cities, but a few simple steps will usually suffice.

1. Keep the body clean! If bodies are released with dried blood on the skin the funeral director will regard your hospital poorly since they must then clean the body themselves.
2. Whenever possible preserve and place long ties on the arteries of the extremities and head, facilitating the process of embalming.
3. Release the body as soon as possible! However, if the requested release time is impossible to meet, call the funeral director, if his name is known, and explain how soon you will be able to release the body.
4. The institution in which you work should provide space where embalming may be done.

CARE OF THE BODY AND RELEASE TO FUNERAL DIRECTOR

The cadaver must always be treated with respect, and blood must not be permitted to dry on the body because it is then more difficult to remove. The incisions will usually be closed by a running "baseball" stitch, and the entire body will be cleaned before release to the undertaker. In order to release the body, proper identification and a properly signed death certificate are required.

It is usually necessary for the funeral director to obtain a burial permit from the local health department, and in order to do so he must have the completed death certificate.

In hospitals with an active resident training

program the viscera are retained for gross organ review unless the autopsy permission specifically directs that they be returned to the body. In non-teaching institutions the organs are usually returned to the body, preferably in plastic bags. This makes the task of the funeral director easier and improves that rapport between pathologist and funeral director which is so easily strained.

Chapter 2

AUTOPSY METHODS AND PROCEDURES

THE AUTOPSY ROOM

THE autopsy room should be so built and equipped as to provide comfortable and sanitary working conditions. It must be properly lit and ventilated. Equipment for storage and preliminary examination of organs should be at hand, and dissecting instruments of all types should be available.

The autopsy room is usually placed on the lower levels of the building adjacent to the mortuary storage areas. This is done so as to facilitate quick and somewhat inconspicuous delivery of the remains to the undertaker once the body has been released from the hospital. It is marked so as to prevent accidental entry of those who have no business in the area.

Adjacent to the autopsy room is a dressing room where the pathologists can change their clothing and store street clothes and possessions while they are in the autopsy room. Ancillary personnel should keep an ample supply of autopsy room clothing available to the pathologist in this area. The type of garment worn by the pathologist varies from hospital to hospital. It is, however, almost always of the surgical uniform type. A shower is available in most recently built dressing rooms. Soaps should be kept available in this area, and it is best that they be of the disinfectant liquid type kept in a container hung over the sink so set up as to release a stream of soap by foot pedal apparatus.

Access to the autopsy room should be available from the dressing room. The dissecting room is best lit with low glare lighting such as suspended or recessed fluorescent lights. The walls are painted with washable paint or covered with tile; the floors are covered with tile or washable concrete and equipped with floor drainage. The placement of the autopsy table will depend upon the construction of the room, its size, shape, and the number of tables present. Any number of autopsy table models are available. Certain basic requirements should be met in the selection of a table. Naturally its dimensions should be such as to accommodate a large cadaver. Those built of reinforced aluminum are easy to care for. Of great importance is the presence of an ample supply of water. Most modern tables are constructed at a slight downward inclination. The cadaver is placed on a perforated metal slab under which a receptable with an active flow of water is present. The final drain from the sink has a filter trap so as to prevent bits of tissue from clogging the pipeline. The table should have a strong suction apparatus fitted with a long plastic pipe with a wide lumen. This should lead to a graduated receptacle so that removed fluids can be accurately measured. Where possible, the table should have an adjustable height. The autopsy room should have opaque or frosted glass windows and should be air-conditioned. Apparatus such as ozone purifiers should be installed to mask or remove occasionally occurring putrescent odors. A cabinet should be kept in the autopsy room containing necessary supplies. These include knives of various sizes, clamps, scissors of several sizes, and equipment available for opening of osseus structures. Wide-mouthed jars containing 10% formalin or Zenker's solution should be available. Smaller bottles for rapid sections should also be available. Five-gallon buckets filled with 20% formalin should be available for brain fixation. All buckets and jars should have labels attached. Iodine solutions and copper sulfate solutions in small quantity should be available for gross testing for the presence of amyloid or fat necrosis as in pancreatitis.

The autopsy room should be equipped with two scales, one large scale for weighing the body while it is on a transportable cart and a pan scale for weighing of organs. A yardstick for determining body length is needed.

Refrigerators for storage of bodies before and after autopsy, until they can be delivered to the undertaker, should be present adjacent to the autopsy room.

A separte dissecting table furnished with an overhead hood with ventilating equipment should be available in the vicinity of the autopsy table.

Organs, once dissected, and sections taken, can be preserved in "Jores" solution for autopsy conference.

Supplies and Equipment

If specimens are to be retained for demonstration at organ review conferences, there must be adequate facilities to preserve them without autolysis. The major options are as follows:

1. Retain the organs in the fresh state in a refrigerator.
2. Retain the tissues in a solution such as Kaiserling's or Jores', both of which provide fixation with less discoloration than formalin. The fixation, however, is not as efficient.
3. After fixation in formalin the coloration of tissues may be slightly restored by placing them in absolute alcohol for several hours.

It may well be that the most important item that an autopsy pathologist possesses is a good knife. One should have at least three different knvies:

1. A scalpel for sharp dissection in removing organs and for dissection of small structures.
2. A medium-sized blade for opening the heart, bivalving the kidney, etc. This should be approximately 12 inches in length.

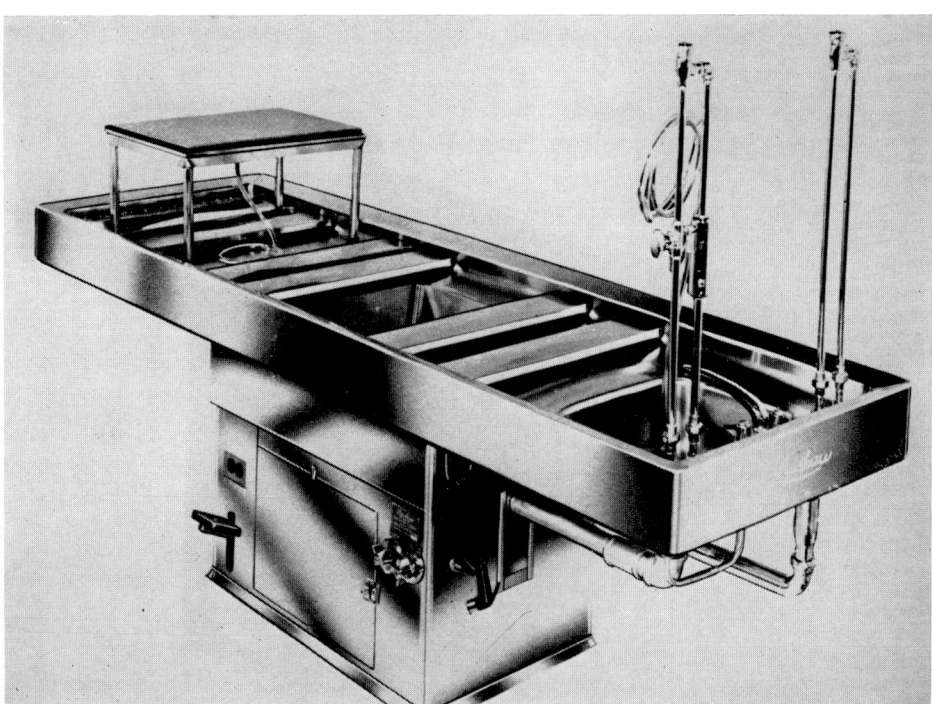

Figure 4. Modern autopsy table with suction apparatus for the removal of fluids. The foot pedal permits height adjustment.

3. A long knife, approximately 18 inches to 24 inches in length for making uniform slices of livers, perfused lungs, and brains.

Aside from the scalpel blades which are of stainless steel and disposable, the other knives are better made of carbon steel because they take and retain a sharper edge than stainless steel.

A good blade sharpener is obviously essential. If an electric sharpener is used, it should be one that can sharpen scissors as well as knives. Scissors should include both straight and curved Mayo scissors and small sharply pointed scissors. An enterotome is also essential. There should be forceps of three kinds, long and short without teeth and short forceps with teeth. There should be long flexible probes as well as short rigid wire probes with a small diameter.

For removing the calvarium and opening the vertebral canal, a vibrating electric saw is used to make the initial incisions avoiding lacerations of the nervous system. Several specially designed hammers and chisels are used to complete the dissection.

A band-saw for the examination of bone lesions is a luxury which is well worthwhile. The vibrating saw distorts the content of the marrow. The band-saw, without the vibrations, does not cause this distortion.

There must also be large and small bottles for fixation of tissues, as well as plastic- or paraffin-coated cardboard buckets for retention of specimens. The fixative's described above must be readily available.

If possible a dictating apparatus with overhead microphone and foot-actuated mechanism is desirable so that dictation of the findings will be concurrent with their discovery.

PREPARATION FOR THE PERFORMANCE OF AN AUTOPSY

The first requirement is that the consent form with any restrictions be reviewed, and that the signature be that of the legal next of kin. It is imperative for the prosector to assure himself at this stage that there are no medicolegal problems that require the case to be reported to the medical examiner or coroner.

In order to perform an autopsy intelligently and to derive the maximum amount of information, it is essential to be fully aware of the clinical history. An autopsy should not be started until the pathologist has read the patient's chart, including laboratory data. Often the nurse's notes and medication record yield

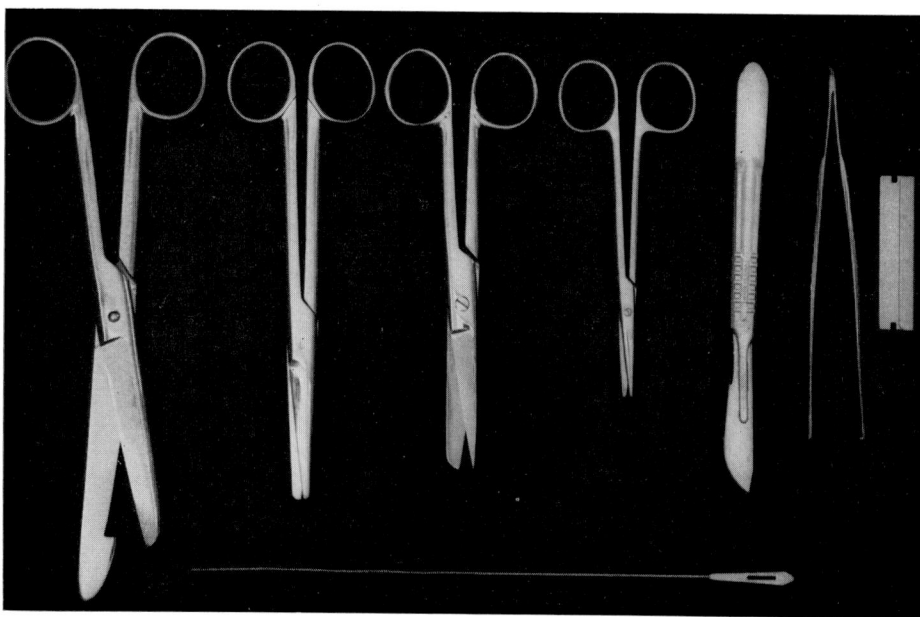

Figure 5. Instruments useful in dissection.

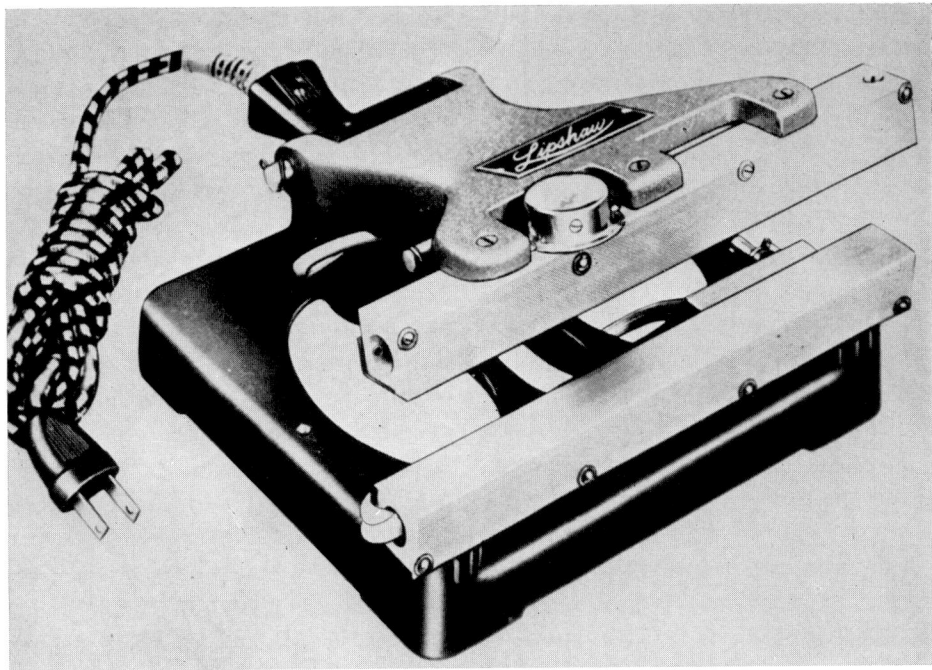

Figure 6. Heat sealing iron for the preservation of tissue in plastic bags.

valuable information not noted in the physician's progress notes. It is highly desirable to have the prosector discuss the case with the physician who attended the patient during life.

The autopsy room attendant should have all instruments and fixative solutions assembled before the start of the autopsy, but these preparations should not unduly delay the start of the autopsy. It is best if an autopsy is performed as soon as possible after death as it may well enable the prosector to obtain more information. In some hospitals autopsies are performed at any time, day or night, when the consent is obtained. In others, autopsies are not performed at night after a predetermined cutoff time unless there are pressing reasons, such as demand for early release of the body or when there is reason to assume that electron microscopical examination or histochemical studies may be needed. The only true advantage to this practice is that it encourages the clinical staff in a teaching hospital to attend the autopsy which they may well be loath to do after attending the patient into the early hours of the morning.

EXTERNAL EXAMINATION

Inspection and palpation are the two principal methods employed in gross anatomic pathology. The body should be placed on the autopsy table after having been weighed. Once placed on the table, its length, crown to heel, should be taken and recorded. The best place to initially record this data is on the toe tag which should be signed by the clinician on the ward. The prosector may at the same time check the tag to ascertain that he is indeed autopsing the proper body. The name on the tag should at this time be checked against the name on the chart. Both the tag and chart name should be checked against the name appearing on the autopsy permit. The name of the nearest of kin on the chart should be checked against that of the person signing the autopsy permit. If any discrepancy exists the autopsy should not proceed until the question is resolved. This moment of caution can spare numerous hours of aggravation.

With the preliminary steps taken and all necessary equipment available, the autopsy may begin. Inspection of the body begins at the head and ends at the toes. During inspection of any given part it should be gently palpated. The hair, color, length, character, e.g. black, long, curly should be noted. The external ear and external auditory canal should be inspected; at the same time the mastoid can be inspected and palpated. The presence of blood secretion should be recorded, as should any deformity or abnormality. The setting of the ears can be noted, low set, etc., as this may be the first clue to the presence of congenital anomalies. The nose is inspected, taking care to examine the septum for possible perforations; any foreign matter present should be described. The eyes are examined. The palpebra, conjunctivae, irides and pupils are inspected and any findings noted. The mouth is inspected. The character of the mucosa is noted. The color of the tongue and its papillations are recorded. In dealing with an unknown body the teeth are carefully inspected and a dental chart is recorded for future use in identification. The body is, of course, fingerprinted for future use in dealing with an unknown person. This is done in large cities by police officers of the missing persons division. The neck is inspected and palpated. The position of the trachea and the size and consistency of the thyroid are noted. The anteroposterior dimensions of the chest are noted, as are the lateral dimensions. The breasts, including areolar and nipples, are inspected. The abdomen is examined; masses, where present, are described. Is the abdomen distended or not? What is the character of the umbilicus? The condition of the genitalia including configuration of pubic hair is recorded. The scrotum is palpated. Are the testis descended? The extremities, particularly the anticubital spaces, are examined. Venepuncture marks or other lesions are noted. The color of the nail-beds is examined. The body is now once more inspected, paying close attention to any skin lesion. Any surgical incisions, recent and remote, are noted and described, paying attention to note the character of the healing which has taken place. The elasticity of the skin is examined, the color of the skin noted, and the distribution and character of the body hair is observed. The distribution of rigor and livor mortis is determined and described. The body is now turned on its side and the back and anus are inspected.

The body should be rinsed by a gentle stream of water prior to making the opening incision. Throughout the course of the autopsy the body and working area should be rinsed at intervals to insure neatness. A sponge should be kept handy and the instruments wiped clean as is needed from time to time during the procedure.

OPENING THE BODY

The external inspection completed, the opening incision can be made. The opening of the scalp and skull will be described in a later chapter.

A block is placed under the shoulders. The prosector, standing at one side of the table, begins by making a Y-shaped incision. The Y-shaped incision can take two forms. This author prefers a shallow Y. With a scalpel in hand an incision in drawn slightly down and forward across the clavicle from one shoulder top to the other. The descending limb of the Y is drawn down the center of the sternum. Once the epigastrium is reached, two fingers are inserted, and the abdominal wall is lifted gently upward. This is done so as to avoid lacerating the abdominal organs with the knife blade. As the incision proceeds downward it passes to one side of the umbilicus so as not to disturb this structure, and below the umbilicus returns to the midline to end at the symphysis pubis. The deep Y begins at one shoulder top, descends lateral to the breast and curves forward along the costal arcade to join the descending limb from the other side at the epigastrium. The abdominal opening proceeds from the epigastrium and is identical in both incisions.

The preliminary incision having been made, it now remains to free the skin of the abdominal and chest walls from their osseous attachments and to free the skin of the neck. The edges of the sternal incision (in the shallow Y) are lifted up with a forceps and dissected free of the underlying bone by a scalpel whose edge the prosector is careful to run along the osseous structures so as not to damage the skin. After an inch or so is freed, the forceps can be put down and the skin placed in gentle traction for for the remainder of dissection by the fingers of the opposite hand. The deep Y is dissected in the same fashion along its margins.

In dissecting the neck, great care should be taken. This part of the dissection should proceed slowly so as not to buttonhole the skin. A light pressure is placed on the blade so as not to damage the structures of the neck. The skin is retracted with four cupped fingers of the opposite hand so as to protect it from the knife blade. The skin of the neck is reflected to the level of the hyoid bone.

Care should be taken to free the skin from the lower costal arcade and to cut its connection at the pubic ramus so as to allow a wide flap. The connection at the pubic ramus is cut without a full thickness incision, cutting only the structures of the inner table of the abdominal wall along the pubic ramus.

THE VIRCHOW METHOD

Examination

With the described skin flaps opened, the internal examination of the body begins. The breasts are examined from within. Four quadrants are incised and the tissue is examined and sections taken. At this point the axillae are examined with special reference to their lymphatic structures. The pectoralis major and minor muscles are incised and examined. The osseous structures of the rib cage are examined, as are their cartilaginous attachments. Prior to opening the rib cage the heights of the diaphragms are noted. The character of the peritoneum is examined. Is it smooth, glistening, and shiny? Or is it dull, gritty, and opaque? The rectus abdominus muscle is in-

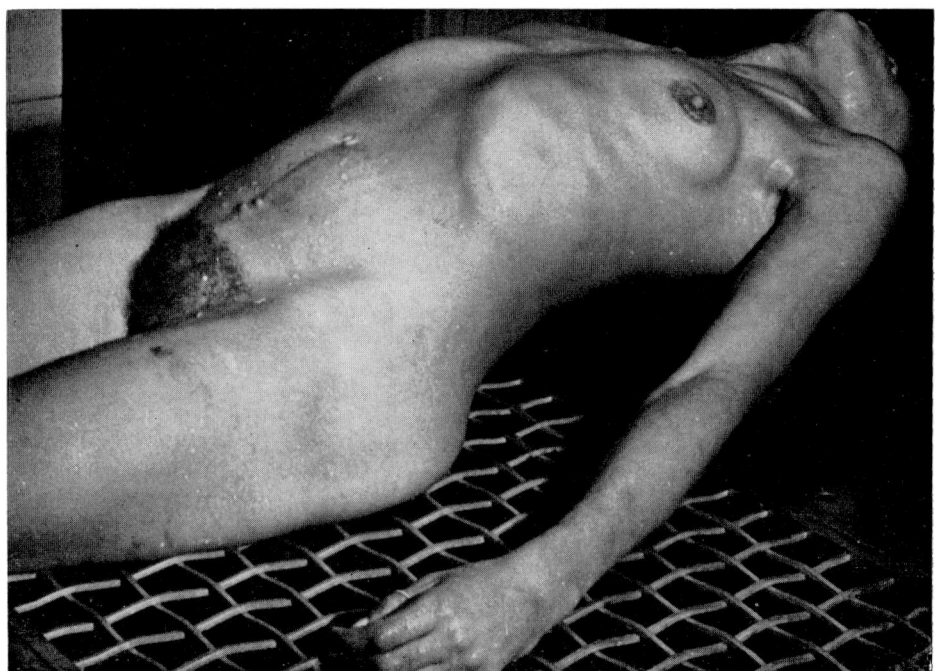

Figure 7

Figures 7, 8, and 9 demonstrate the opening of the body.

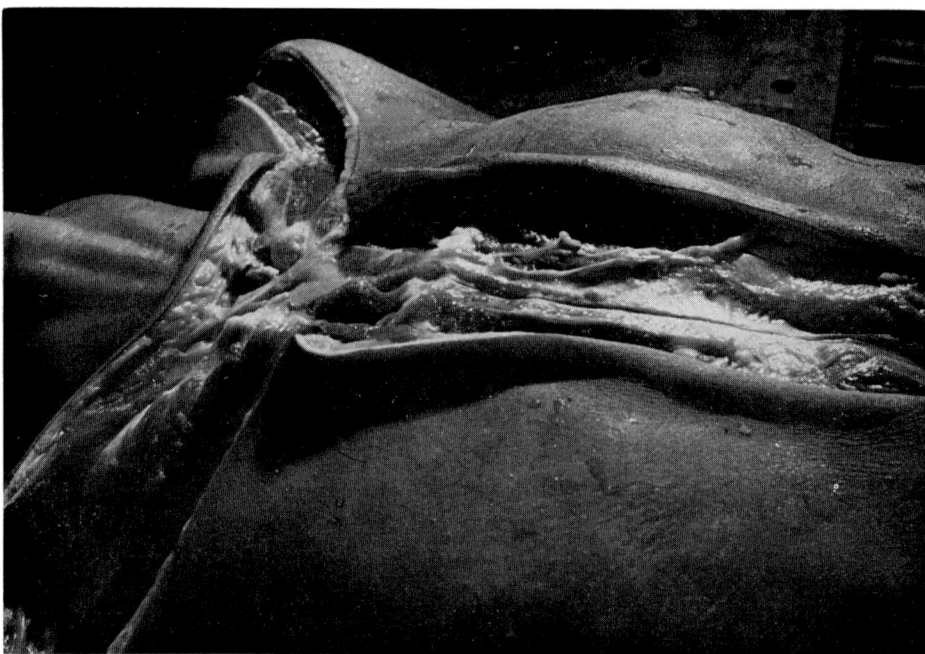

Figure 8

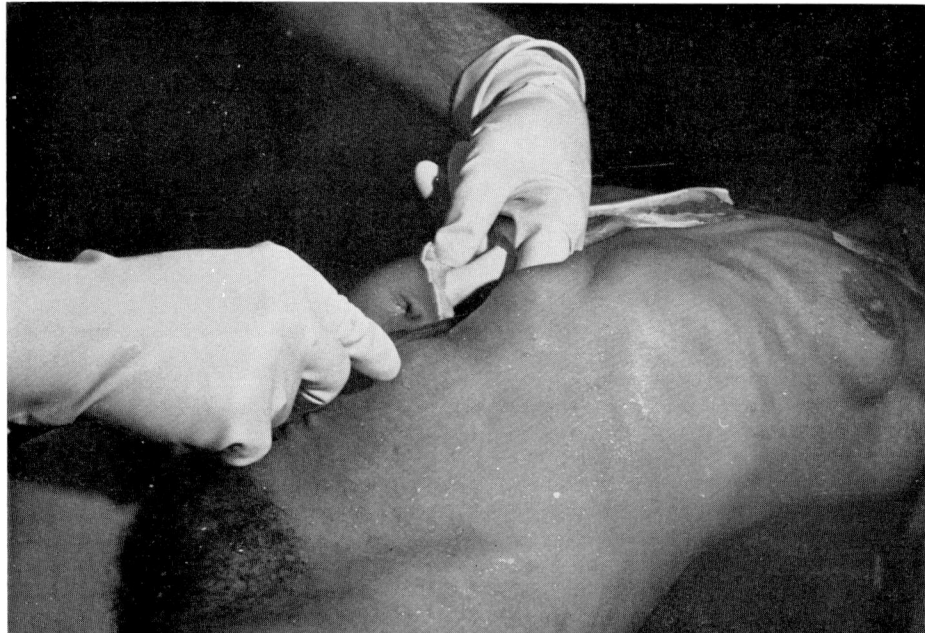

Figure 9

cised and examined. The situs of the abdominal organs is described; the presence of fluids in the abdominal cavity is determined, its character described and its quantity measured. The greater omentum is now examined and cut free. The small intestine is reflected and spread out while still attached so that its mesentery can be evaluated. Mesenteric vessels are incised at various points for examination. The portal vein is located, traced to its entrance at the liver, incised, examined, and cut free. The ligament of Treitz is located and clamped. This author finds it easier to use two 6-inch clamps than to tie off with string. The intestine between the clamps is cut, and the intestine is run along a long sharp knife which is manipulated in a back and forth sawing motion. Once the ileocecal area is reached, the caecum is examined and the presence, position, and form of the appendix is determined. The ascending colon is lifted forward gently to the hepatic flexure which is then examined. The transverse colon is similarly lifted forward on its mesentery; the splenic flexure is examined as is the descending

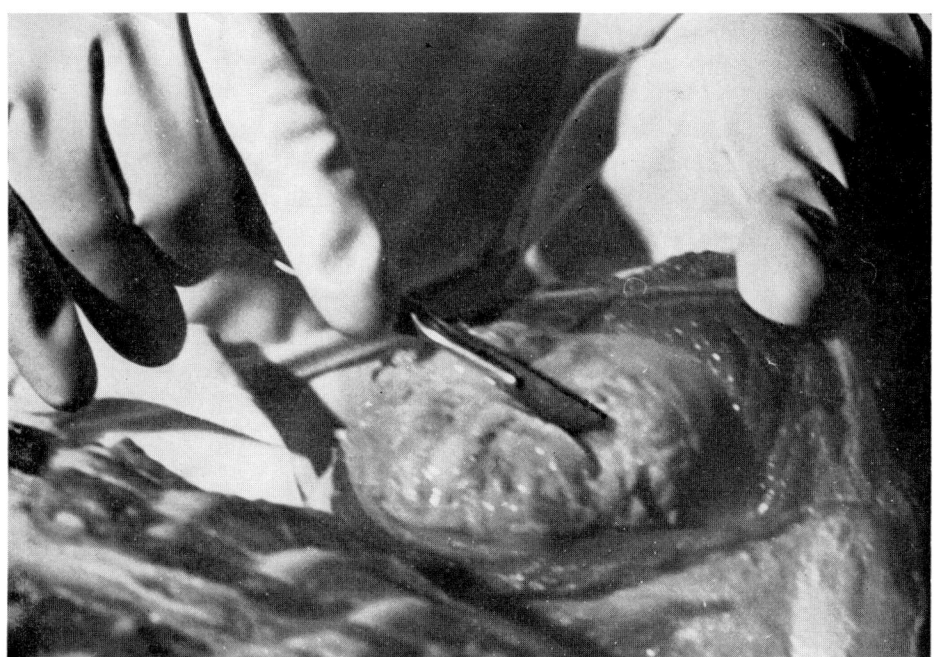

Figure 10. Four quadrant sampling of breast at autopsy.

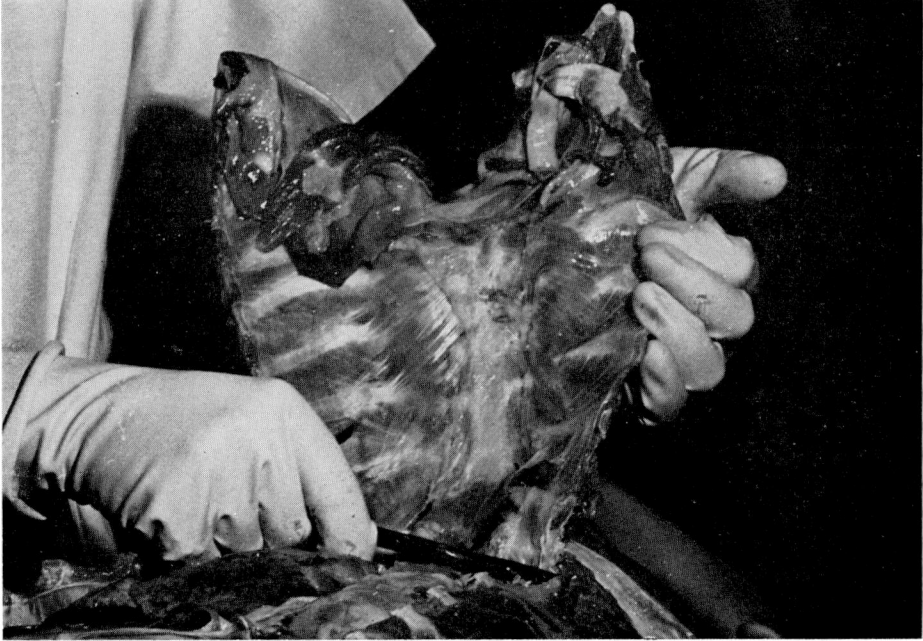

Figure 11. Removal of the breast plate.

colon. With the mesenteries loose, the same sawing motion is employed with the knife, and the colon is exteriorized. At the rectosigmoid junction two additional 6-inch clamps are applied and the connection severed. The distal portion for the time being remains *in situ*. The colon is placed in a pan for future examination.

We now proceed to open the thoracic cavity. The standard method usually employed is to separate the clavicle from the sternum by dissection with a scalpel. The author prefers not to sacrifice that articulation, but rather to keep it intact so that he can retain an entire articulation for microscopic examination. The dissection, therefore, proceeds by beginning to separate the rib cage lateral to the articulations. An electrical saw is used. About 2 inches lateral to the articulation the clavicle and ribs are cut to the costal arcades. The bones, having been separated, the lower portion of the rib cage is reflected upward and separated from its soft tissue connections by dissection with a scalpel. Care is taken to direct the scalpel blade against the bone so as not to harm underlying tissue. With the rib cage opened, the inspection and *in situ* evaluation of the chest is begun. The visceral and parietal pleura are examined. Are they smooth, glistening, and shiny? Or are they dull, gritty, and opaque? The presence of fibrothorax is determined and described. Fluids present are described, removed, and measured. The ribs are examined, including examination of the removed chest plate. At this point, one sternoclavicular joint may be sectioned with the electric saw and placed in the fixative bottle. Examination of the mediastinum should now be carried out. The character of the pericardium is noted. When present, the thymus should be removed and weighed. Sections should be taken. The great vessels are traced *in situ*; their courses and relationships are noted. Following inspection of the great vessels, the aortic branches are traced into the neck. In so doing, one places slight traction on the carotids so that they are displaced laterally. They are tied off at the root of the neck and severed below the ties. The thyroid is palpated, as is the trachea, hyoid bone, and floor of the mouth. Before proceeding with the dissection, the thyroid arteries are located. These give off small branches to the parathyroids which can be located *in situ* on the posterior medial surface of the thyroid and removed before the prosector causes major structural alterations. To facilitate this the thyroid lobes are reflected medially.

Evisceration

Evisceration begins at the neck and proceeds in a caudal direction. The neck block is removed together with the tongue. A long sharp knife is placed at the angle of the mandible and introduced upward. The knife is then brought with its cutting margin leading around to the opposite mandibular angle. Two fingers are introduced through the floor of the mouth, and traction is placed on the tongue which is brought down underneath the mandible. As the tongue is displaced forward, the hyoid trachea, pharynx, and esophagus are cut free of their posterior connections. The tongue is examined in its relationships and severed from the lower tissue mass just above the hyoid. It is placed in a pan for future examination. The hyoid is cut free and also retained. At this point the prosector will examine the course and relationships of the esophagus. It may then be severed and a clamp placed at its upper end to facilitate later dissection. Alternately, the esophagus can be left in place for later dissection. The epiglottis, thyroid, and trachea are severed just above the carina and retained for later examination. The prosector might elect when dealing with disease of the respiratory tract to leave the tracheobronchial tree intact for formalin inflation and fixation with the lung block with which it may be electively removed retaining connections.

Evisceration of the chest organs may now begin. The pericardium is opened and described. Fluid contained in the pericardial cavity is described and measured. The ascending aorta and arch are examined. The aorta is clamped just below the arch and severed. The pulmonary artery is opened *in situ* and examined for thromboemboli. The pulmonary veins

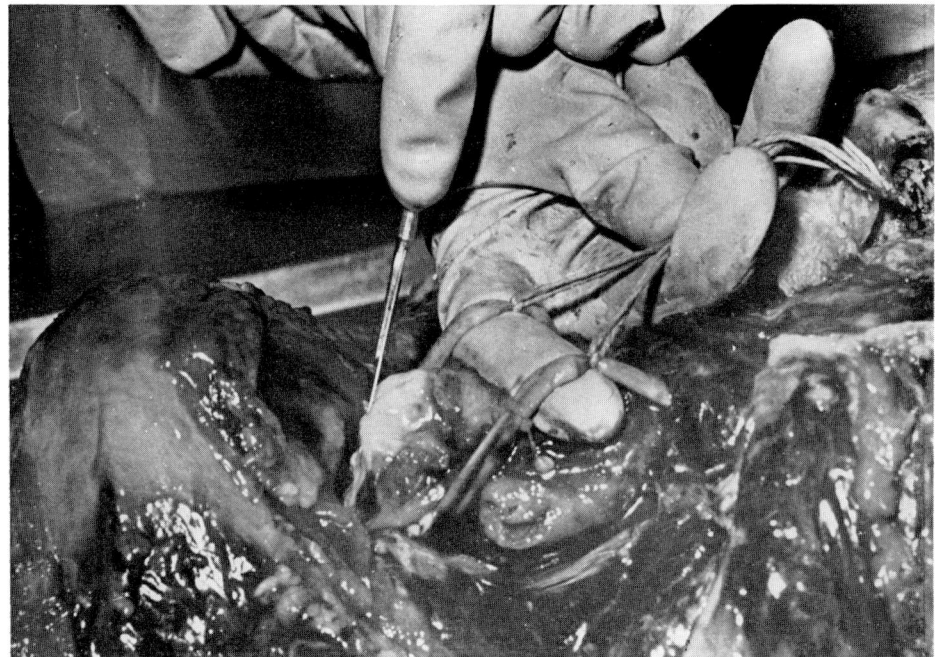

Figure 12

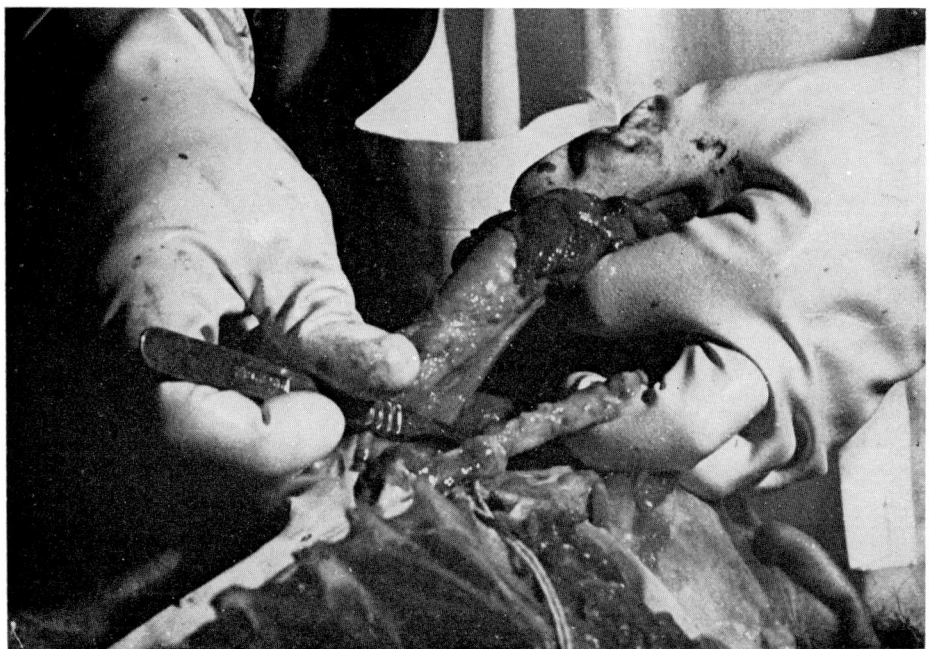

Figure 13

Figures 12 and 13 demonstrate the dissection and removal of the neck block.

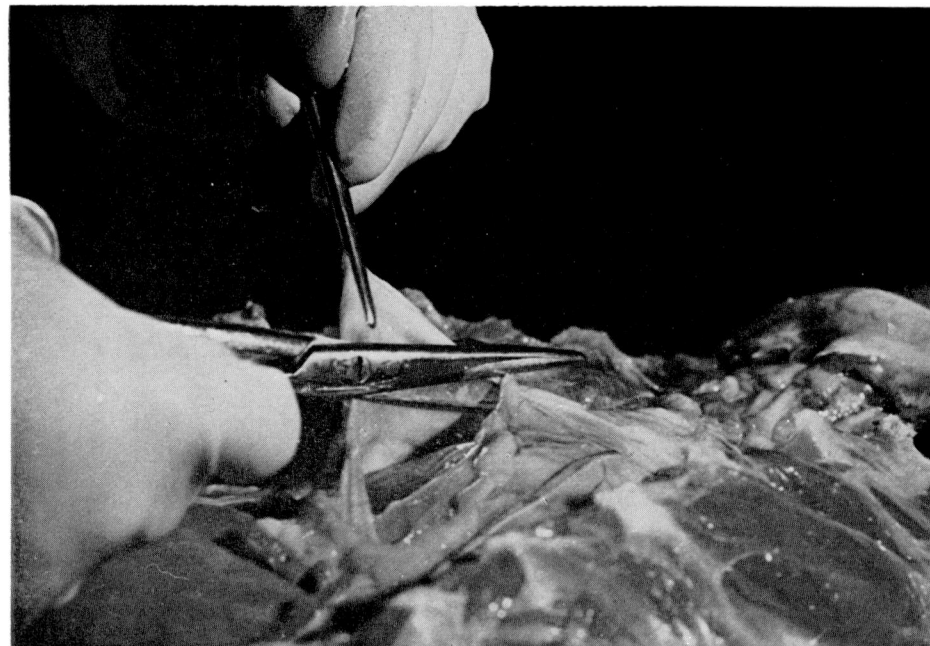

Figure 14. Opening of the pericardium.

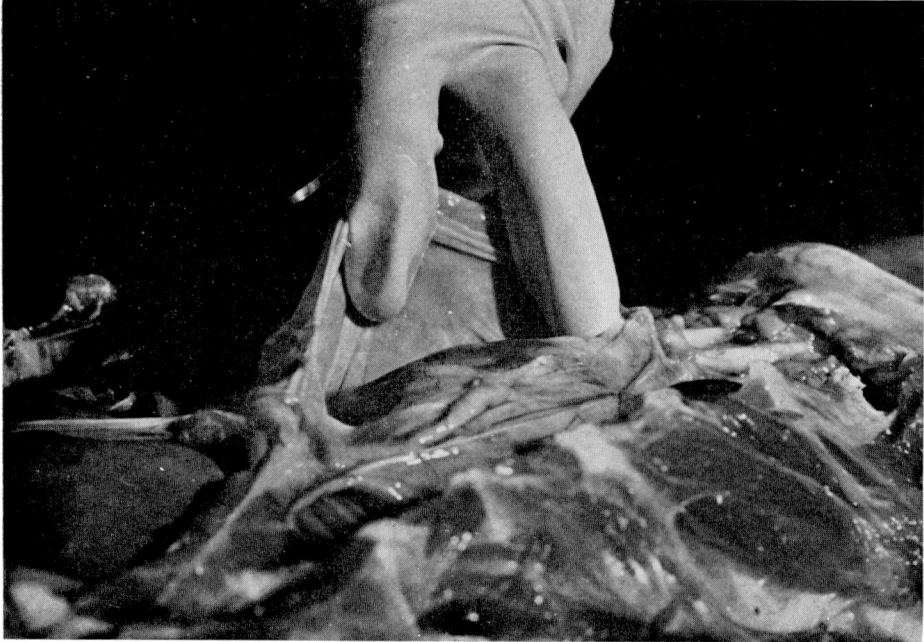

Figure 15. Inspection of the pericardial sac.

are examined as they enter the left atrium and as far as possible traced back to the lungs. The superior vena cava is traced to its entry into the right atrium. The dissection continues at this point into the inferior vena cava as it passes up from the diaphragm. This author prefers at this point to follow the inferior vena cava into the abdomen, tracing and opening it along its entire course and relationship into the abdominal cavity. At this point the prosector returns to the chest and by cutting along the pulmonary arteries severs this connection. The vena cava

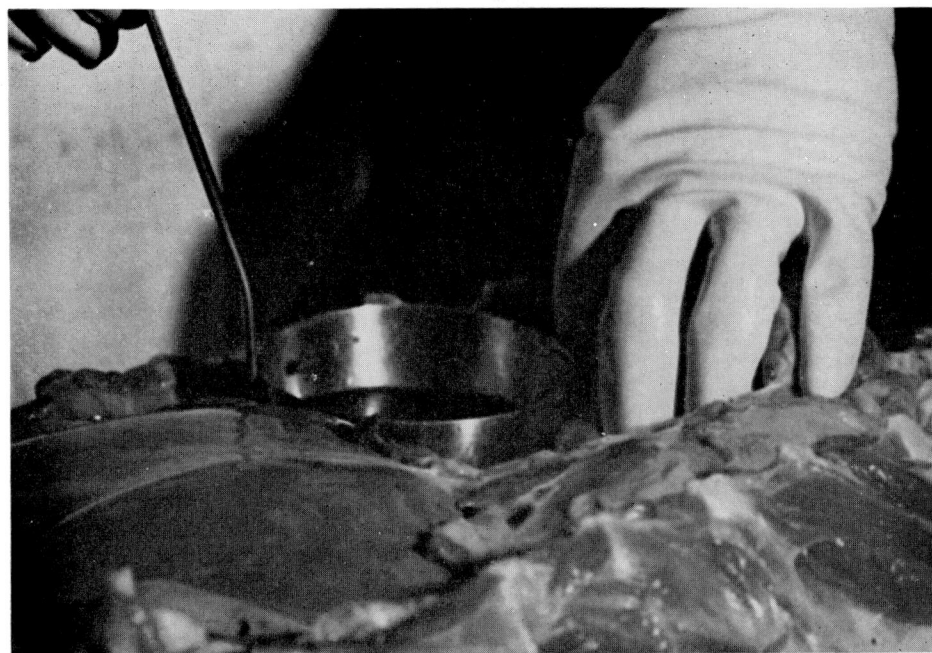

Figure 16. Removal of fluid from the pericardium.

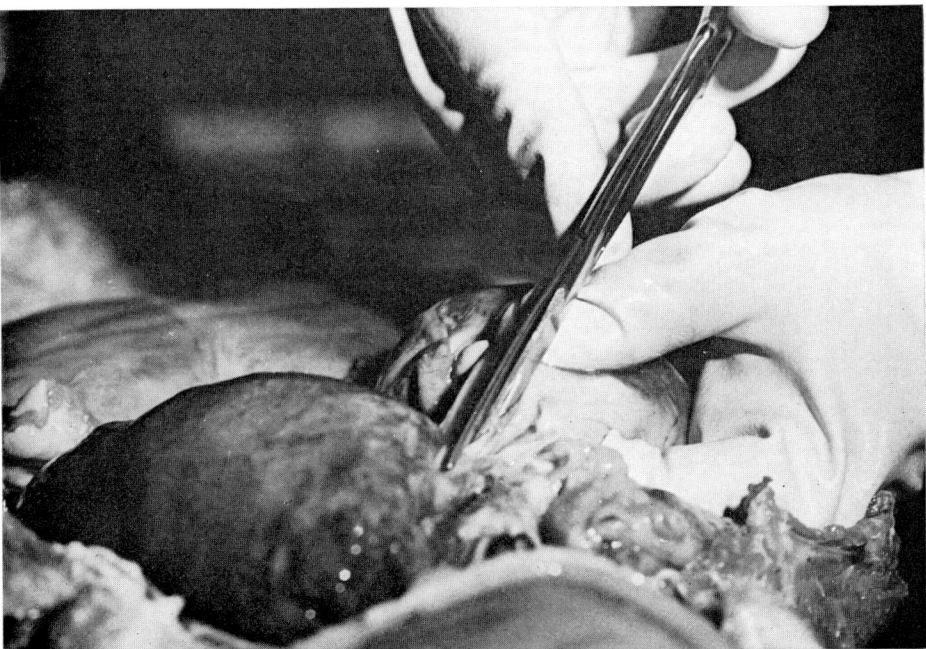

Figure 17. *In situ* opening of the pulmonary artery.

is severed; the heart is then reflected upward and the pulmonary veins are cut. At this point the heart comes free with the aortic arch. The prosector may now proceed to remove the lungs. One hand is placed in the hilum of the lung; the lung is reflected laterally and the hilar structures are cut. The same procedure is followed for the opposite lung. Where the trachea has been maintained in its connections with the bronchi, it is directed forward and cut from behind to free the entire block.

We now proceed to the abdominal eviscera-

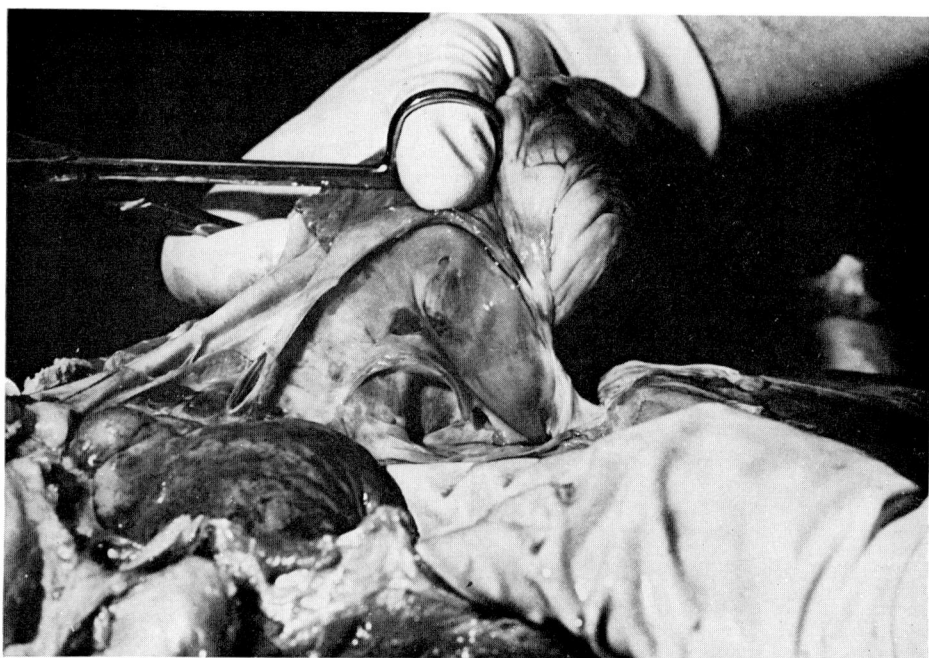

Figure 18. Opening of the Vena Cava.

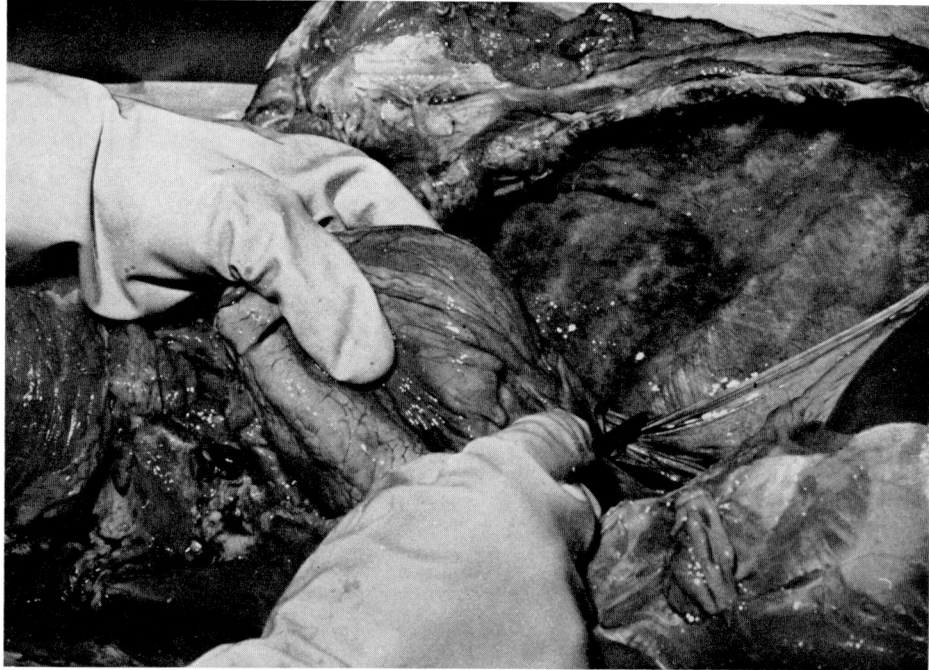

Figure 19. Removal of the heart from the mediastinum.

tion. In the abdomen the splenic artery is traced to the hilum of the spleen, examining the pancreas as this is done. The spleen is lifted anterolaterally and severed from its connection. The liver can now be examined *in situ* prior to its removal. It is lifted backward so as to show the gallbladder, which is freed of its bed by sharp dissection. The hepatic and common ducts are cut free at the same time. The liver is repositioned in its anatomical position. The falciform and coronary ligaments are cut and the liver is lifted free.

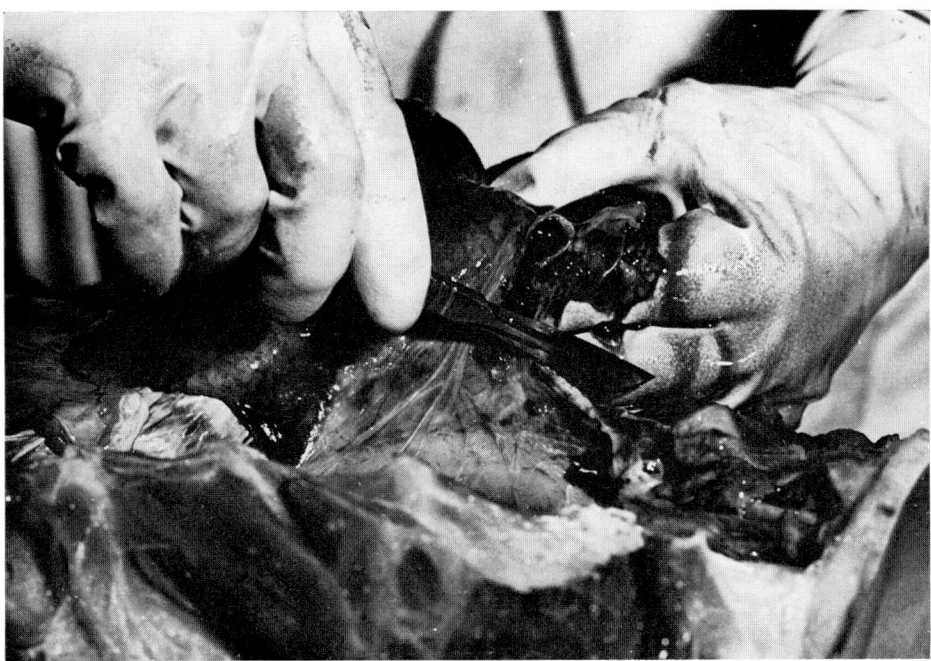

Figure 20. Removal of lung.

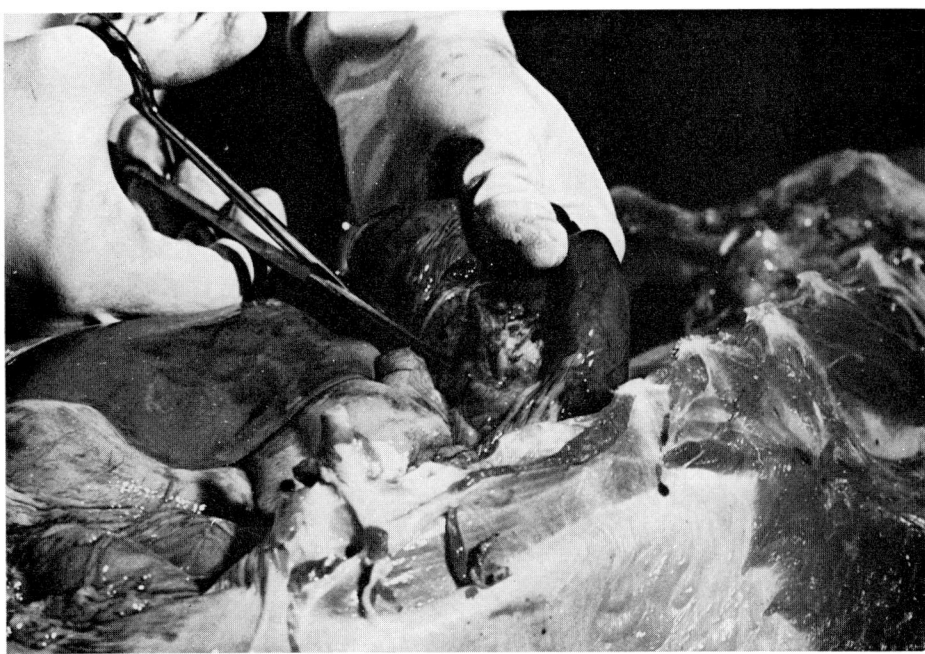

Figure 21. Removal of the spleen.

The intestines are removed in the following manner: the ligament of Treitz is located and ligated. Cutting between the ligatures, the small intestine is removed by employing a sawing motion with a long knife against the mesenteric border. When the large intestine is reached, it is freed in the same manner along its course. The rectosigmoid junction is ligated and the intestine is freed. The remaining portion is removed with the pelvic organs.

The diaphragm is now opened from its ventral margin to the esophageal hiatus. The

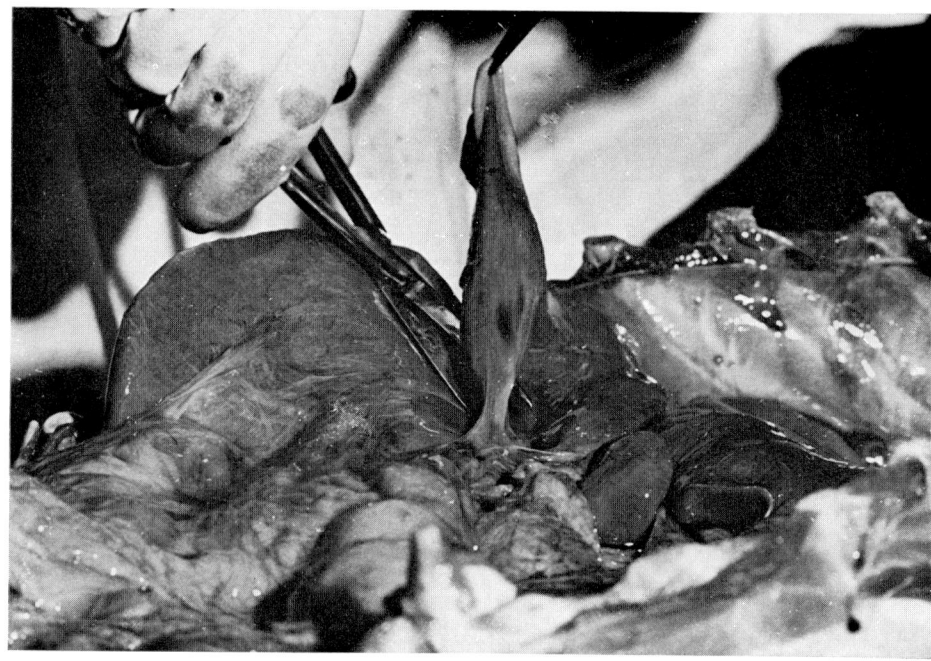

Figure 22

Figures 22 and 23 demonstrate the removal of the liver.

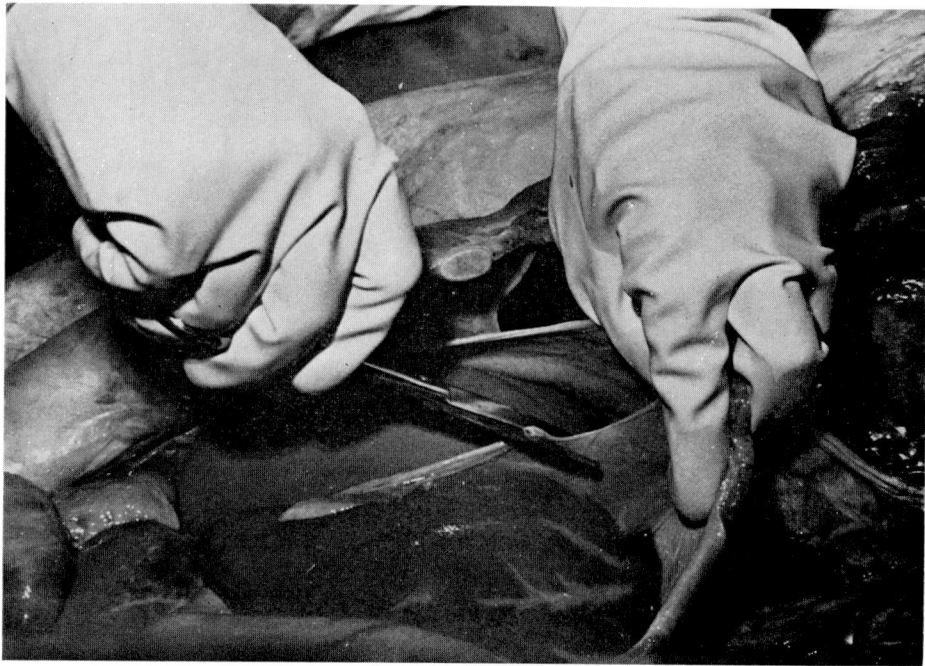

Figure 23

esophagus is reflected forward into the abdomen. Alternately, where the superior esophageal connection has not been severed, the stomach, duodenum, gallbladder, and pancreas are lifted forward, cut from their inferior connective tissue and vascular connections and removed, passing into the chest where the esophagus is severed from above.

The prosector now returns to the chest. The aorta is located and an *in situ* opening is carried

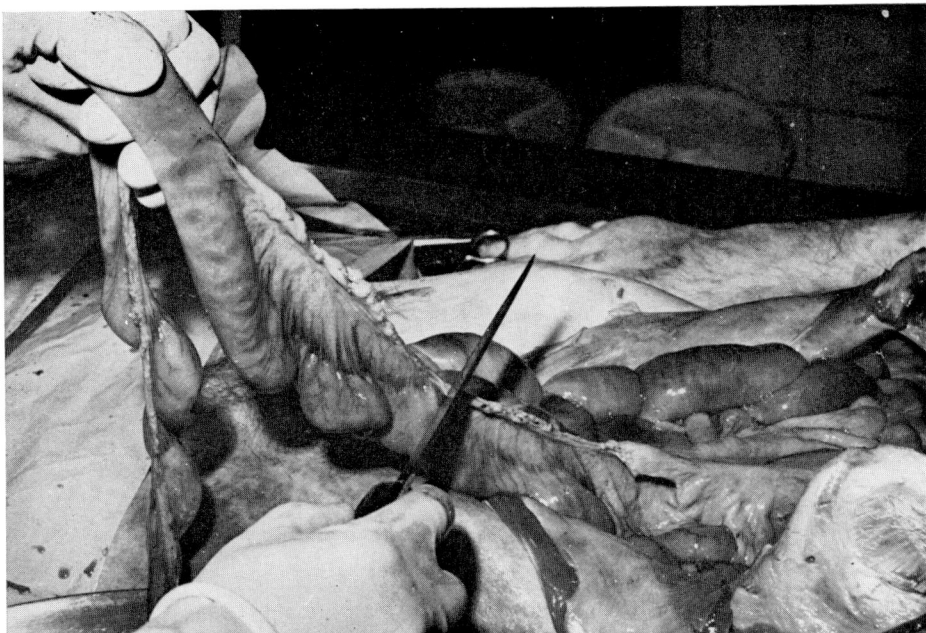

Figure 24. Removal of the intestine.

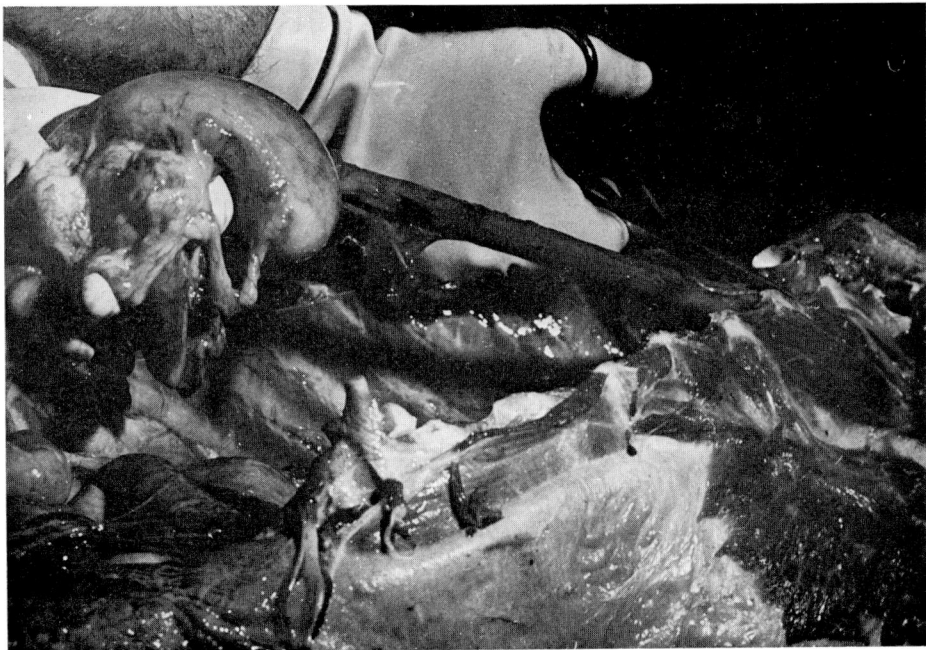

Figure 25. Removal of the stomach and esophagus.

out by placing the superior end under slight traction and opening the ventral surface with a scissor passing through the diaphragm and continuing down to the iliac arteries. The renal arteries are traced and opened. Once examined, the renal arteries may be severed from the aorta. The kidneys are palpated and the adrenals are located by palpation. They are lifted by a forceps and separated from the renal surfaces.

The kidneys are lifted anterolaterally; in so doing, the ureters are loosened. They are then

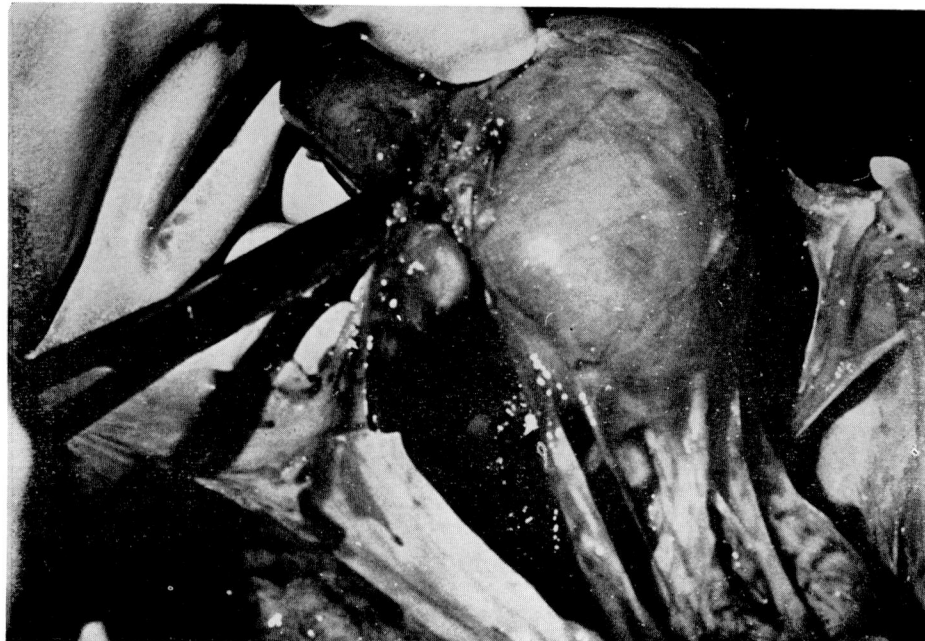

Figure 26. Dissection of the renal vessels prior to dissection of the kidney.

freed by manual dissection along their course. With the renal hilum held in the palm of the hand, the concavity of the perirenal fat pad is incised and pealed away from the renal surfaces along with the capsules. This tissue mass is freed from around the kidney by a scissors. If the incision of the renal fat pad has been properly delivered through the kidney, it will split the pelvis at midpoint. A sharp, narrow-bladed scissor is used, and the ureters are opened along their entire course to their entrance point into the bladder at the trigone. The ureters may now be severed or, if desired, maintained in their connections with the bladder.

It will be remembered at this point that the rectum and bladder, the prostate in the case of a male, the uterus in the case of a female, and adnexae have not been removed. The bladder is freed from its anterior connections by manual blunt dissection. The rectum, uterus or prostate, and the bladder are surrounded by the entire hand and with a long sharp knife separated from their pelvic connections. This is facilitated by placing the organs in firm upward traction. Once the inferior connections are severed, the rectum is dissected free of its posterior connection by a scalpel. The organs may now be removed as a block. The aorta may now be removed from its posterior connections by sharp dissection.

The vertebral column can now be examined and a block taken for evaluation of the marrow and bone. This author prefers to take a section of bone after the spinal cord is removed.

Where no muscle disease exists we take routnie muscle and nerve sections from the psoas area. Where disease exists, as many muscle groups as is possible are sampled.

With the evisceration complete the prosector now reexamines the osseous structures by inspection and palpation prior to beginning the individual organ dissections.

Where emboli are found, the popliteal and femoral vessels are opened and sampled.

The testes are removed by entering the scrotal sac from above the pubic ramus. With the other hand the testes are delivered upward through the sac. They are now lifted out with the spermatocord and freed.

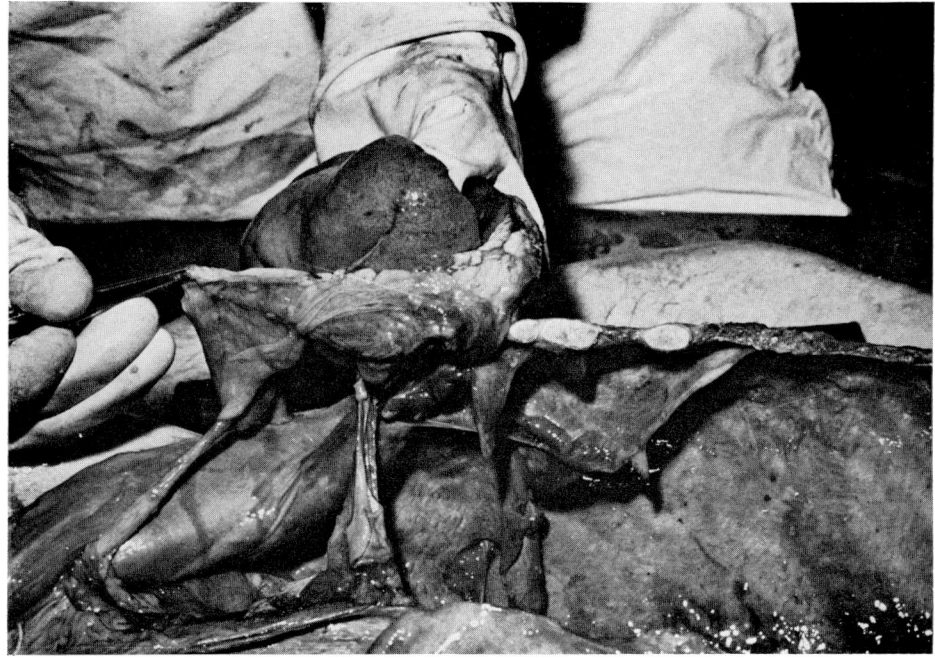

Figure 27

Figures 27 and 28 demonstrate the *in situ* dissection of the kidney.

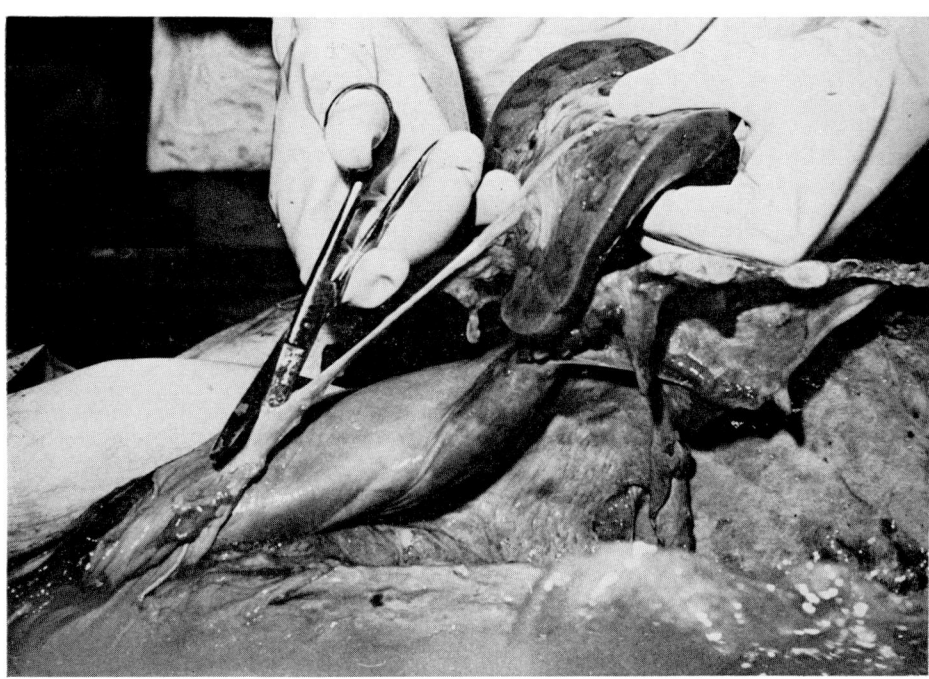

Figure 28

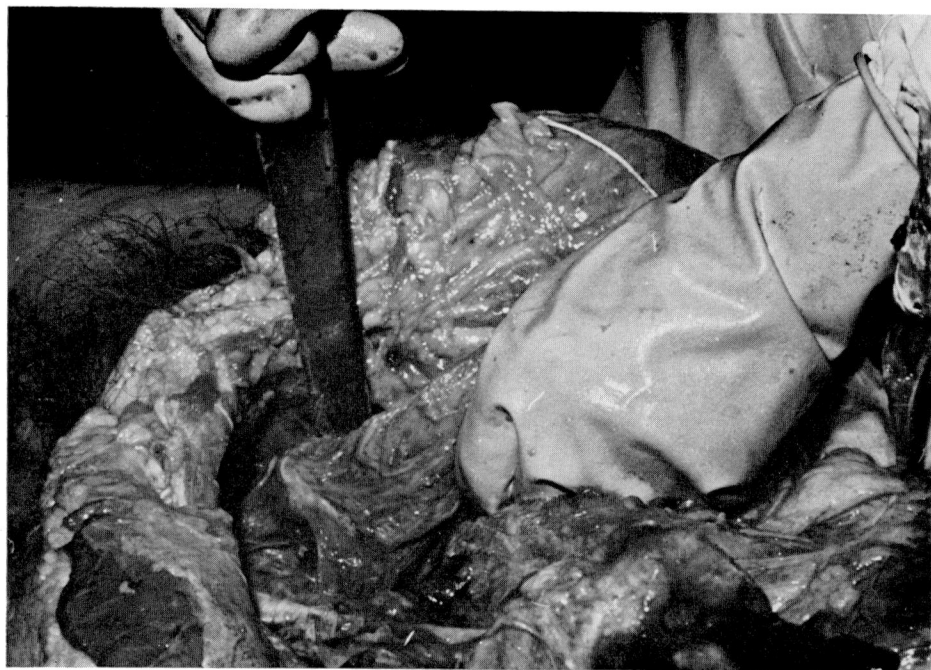

Figure 29. Removal of the pelvic block.

THE ROKITANSKY METHOD

The so-called Rokitansky or modified Rokitansky procedure is the method of evisceration most often used at our hospital. This method has the distinct advantage of retaining the relationships of the various organs, particularly of the vascular systems of the liver, upper gastrointestinal tract, and kidneys. Single organ dissection often masks this relationship.

After opening the body as described earlier and carefully examining the organs *in situ*, the removal of the viscera begins.

The superior extent of dissection is often determined by clinical indications. Optimally, for complete examination, the oral and pharyngeal structures will be examined. This procedure involves removal of the oropharyngeal wall and tongue by the passage of a scalpel along the inner surface of the mandible and the anterior surface of the cervical portion of the vertebral column. When performing this procedure the nasopharyngeal recess (fossa of Rosenmüller) and uvula should be inspected and additional material removed should any abnormalities be detected. In many cases there is no indication of disease in the oral cavity or oropharynx. If this be the case, the superior limit of dissection may routinely be made just above the epiglottis by a tranverse incision. Using traction on the larynx or supralaryngeal tissues, the organs are lifted from the vertebral column with careful sharp dissection.

When the diaphragm is reached it must be cut about its circumference and its posterior border incised with care to avoid injuring the esophagus and blood and lymphatic vessels adjacent to the vertebral column.

Continuing traction on the upper portion of the block, the abdominal block is removed with incision of the posterior attachments to the vertebral column and lateral incision of the peritoneum into the pelvis with care not to transect the ureters.

At this point the pelvic block may be removed in one of two ways. The usual procedure is to grasp the pelvic organs in one hand and to free their posterior and lateral attachments by blunt dissection. The rectum is then ligated to avoid fecal contamination. A large knife is then passed along the symphysis pubis, removing the pelvic mass. Alternately, the pelvic block may be removed by an oval incision in the peritoneum, including anus, vagina and urethra in females, and anus in males.

Removal of the entire penis is usually not feasible. However, should examination of the urethra or glans penis be indicated with a combination of blunt and sharp dissection, the shaft and glans may be removed by separation from the overlying skin. This may be removed *en bloc* with the remainder of the pelvic block by inserting a blade beneath the symphysis pubis and making a circumferential incision.

At this point, the block having been removed, it is examined from the posterior surface. As stated, the advantage of en bloc evisceration is preservation of relationships, particularly of vascular structures. Within the thorax, the thoracic duct and aorta may be identified from the posterior surface. Within the abdomen, the aorta and vena cava are identified. The vena cava, which lies posteriorly, is opened for its entire length, including the iliac veins, taking care not to sever the right renal artery which passes posterior to the vena cava. The aorta is opened along its length including the proximal portions of the iliac arteries. The renal arteries are opened and the orifices of the celiac axis, superior mesenteric, and inferior mesenteric arteries inspected. If there be no disease noted in the renal arteries, they may be transected, facilitating examination of the renal veins. Otherwise, they may be carefully dissected from the underlying ureters and veins. The renal veins are then opened and examined. The aorta is transected at the diaphragm and reflected downward. The portal vein is located and is opened along with the superior mesenteric and splenic veins. At this point the block may be divided for easier handling and examination of individual organs.

The esophagus is separated from the adjoining chest organs and reflected to the diaphragm. The chest organs are then separated from the block by an incision along the superior surface of the diaphragm. The thoracic aorta is then reflected superiorly, and the heart and aorta are easily separated from a block composed of pharynx, larynx, trachea, and lungs by severing the pulmonary arteries and veins.

The adrenal glands are identified and excised. The kidneys are removed from the abdominal block by a combination of blunt and sharp dissection. They are then removed in continuity with ureters, carefully separating these structures from the adjacent fibroadipose tissue, the urinary bladder and urethra, including penis, if this has been excised. In the case of females, the uterus, ovaries, fallopian tubes, and vagina are then separated from the block.

The gallbladder is dissected away from the liver and preserved with the stomach, duodenum and pancreas. The liver is removed. The spleen is separated from the pancreas. At this point fragments of adherent fibroadipose tissue may be removed and each of the separate blocks dissected as described for individual organs. Removal of the testes, vertebral bone, and brain is conducted as described in the section on removal of the individual organs.

INDIVIDUAL ORGAN DISSECTIONS

Regardless of whether the Virchow or Rokitansky methods have been employed in the evisceration, the method of individual organ dissection remains the same.

Tongue

The tongue, having been previously severed from its lower connections, may now be studied. The tongue is placed in its anatomic position and inspected from back to front. The lingual tonsils, which lie laterally, are noted and their size evaluated. They may be excised for section if this is seen to be necessary. Similarly, the small mucous glands are evaluated. The vallate, filiform, and fungiform papillae, are examined.

Areas of leukoplakia are excised and saved for study.

The tongue is now incised in steps from back to forward, and the disposition of the muscular fascicles is examined. Small tumours, where found, are excised. The submaxillary glands removed in the dissection are studied by gross examination and section.

The Hyoid Bone

The hyoid bone is now examined. To facilitate this examination the connected soft tissue must be dissected away. Care must be taken in this dissection so as not to produce artefactual fracture. The body, and greater and lesser horns of the hyoid are examined and described.

The Thyroid Gland

The inexperienced pathologist might encounter difficulty in interpretation of his thyroid dissection. The dissection itself is relatively simple. The skeletal portion of the laryngeal block is placed face down. The thyroid is then removed by forceps and scalpel dissection. The forcep places light traction on the gland, and it is dissected away from the underlying bone with the knife blade oriented against the bone. This continues in a back to front dissection until the anterior midline is reached. At this point the prosector returns to the opposite side and repeats the procedure. This dissection completed, the gland is placed face up, and sections are made from the upper to the lower poles through the entire gland.

The gland may show various alterations depending upon its functional state. It is, however, usually dark, red-brown, and contains glistening colloid material. The right and left lobes are joined in the midline by an isthmus which is missing in 50 percent of the cases. Accessory thyroid tissue may be seen in the midline along the course of the thyroglossal duct. Accessory thyroid tissue is sometimes found in the level between the suprahyoid region and the aortic arch. Areas of nodularity, tumour, and fibrosis should, of course, be sectioned. The gland should be described as to size, form, color, consistency, and relation to surrounding tissue. Surrounding lymph nodes, where found, should be sectioned and retained for study.

The Tracheolaryngeal Block

The tracheolaryngeal block is opened by placing the block face down and opening it with a scissor through the membranous portions. Light pressure placed on the superior thyroid horns allows the thyroid cartilage to be spread, facilitating examination. The epiglottis is examined; the mucosa is evaluated as to congestion and edema. Any specifically abnormal areas are sectioned. The epiglottis is then depressed to allow examination of the vallecula. The ventricular band and true cord are sectioned. This is done by a single section taken in an up down direction so as to contain the ventricle itself.

The osseous structures are examined and described. The thyroid cartilage, cricoid cartilage, arytenoid cartilages, and the lumina are examined and described, as are the interposed membraneous structures.

The Lungs

The lungs, having been removed, are individually weighed and recorded. The lung is now placed in its anatomic position on the dissecting table. The pleura are examined. Are they smooth, glistening, and shiny? Or are they dull, gritty, and opaque? The presence of exudates or adhesions should be described. Are exudates fibrinous or hemorrhagic purulent or serous? The subpleural lymphatics are examined. Are they clear? or do they contain tumour material?

The lung is now examined by light palpation. The lung is gently passed between the cupped fingers, and areas of consolidation or granularity are noted. An infarct found in the lung may be described as "a firm, well-demarcated wedged-shaped structure," which is brown, dry, granular on cut section, and surrounded by a hyperemic halo. The lobar divisions are examined, including the interlobar fissures.

The lung is now turned with its hilar surface face up. The anatomic relationships of the veins, arteries, and bronchi are examined. Hilar lymph nodes are removed, sectioned, and described. It is advisable to perform all organ

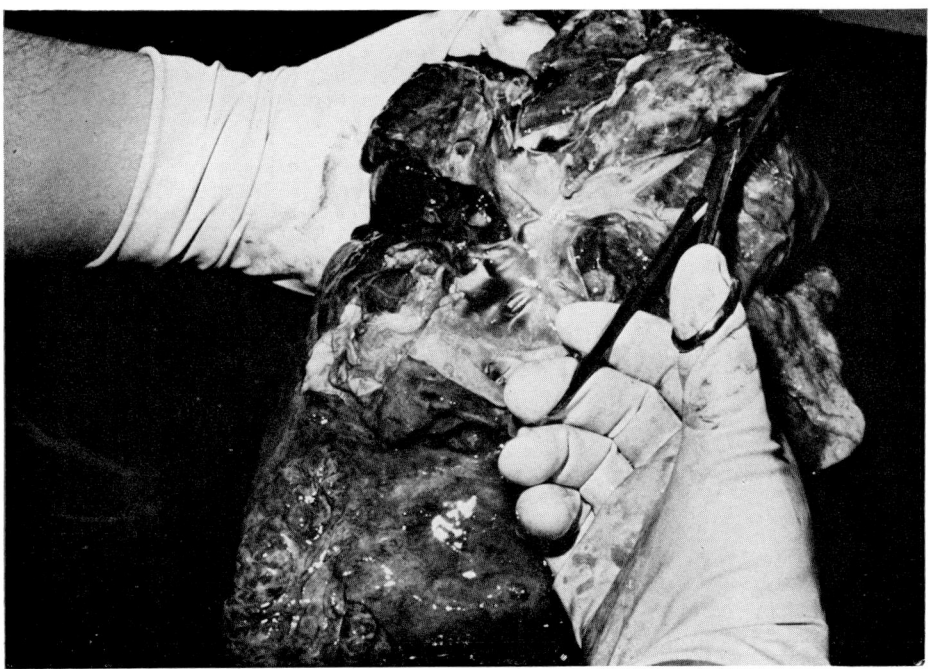

Figure 30

Figures 30, 31, and 32 demonstrate the dissection of the lung.

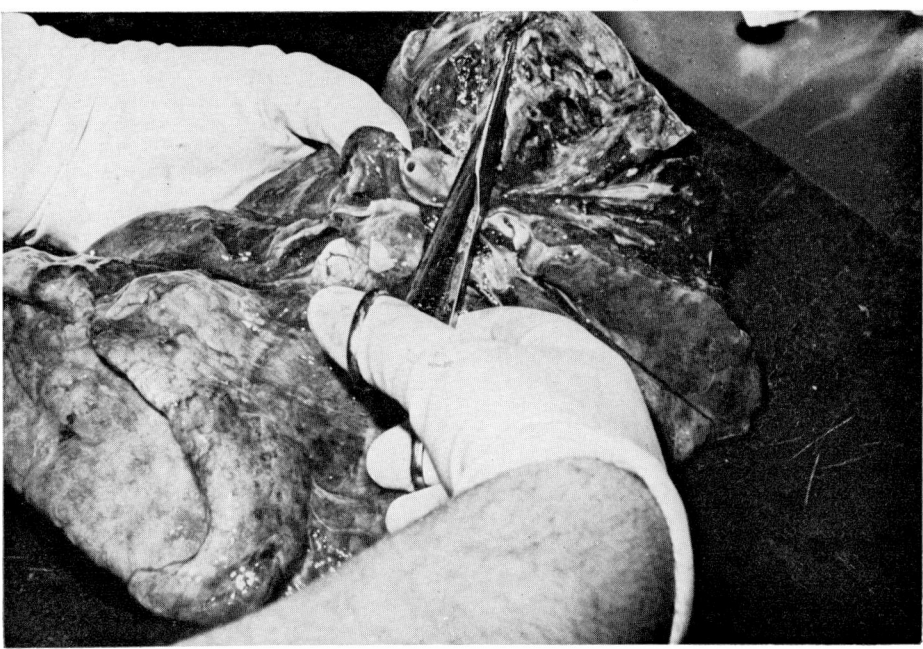

Figure 31

dissections with a steady stream of cool water available to remove fluids as they occur so as to prevent obscuring the structures to be described. With a sharp, long-nosed scissors the pulmonary arteries and veins are opened; their course and relationships are noted. The presence of pulmonary atherosclerosis is noted, and the extent of its distribution throughout the vascular tree is described. The bronchi are opened and the character of their mucosa is

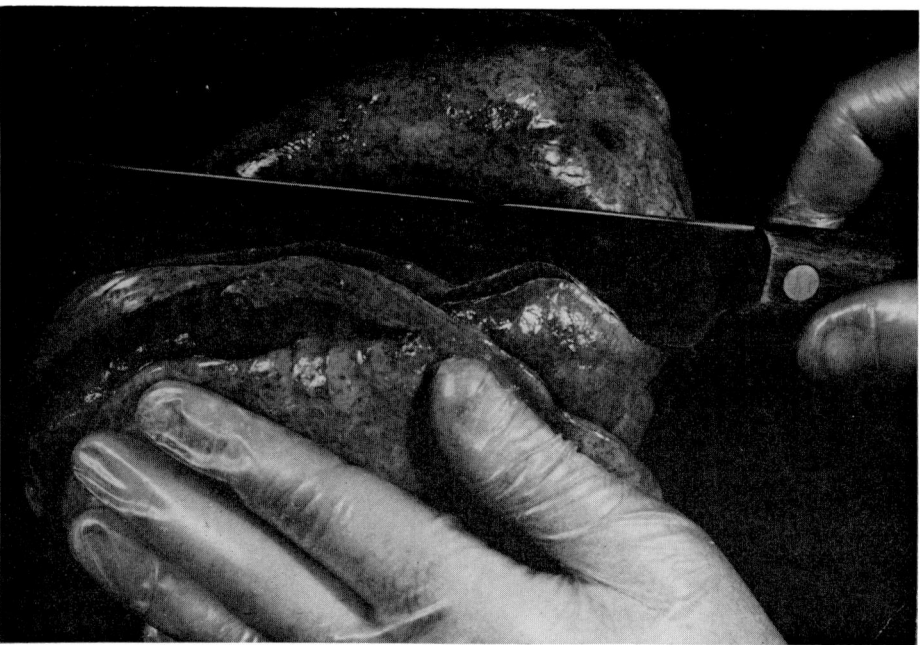
Figure 32

described. The thickness of their walls is noted. The luminal content is examined and described. Special note should be taken of the relationships of the bronchi, one to the other. Are they tubular? Do they aggregate together? Are they particularly dilated? Do they lead into a cavity? Is tumour present?

The lung is now returned to its nonhilar surface. With a long knife the parenchyma is incised from apex to base. Examination of the parenchyma may now begin. Methodical examination from apex to base is advised. In examining the apex, care should be taken to find possible evidence of old or active tuberculosis. Cavities, where found, should be described as to size, form, and capsule. Is material present in the cavity? What is its quantity, color, and consistency? Is the cavity wall smooth surfaced, or is it rough? Are blood vessels noted in the wall? Can a point of hemorrhage be found?

The parenchyma is described. Is it well aerated, elastic, fluffy, and crepitant? Is it poorly aerated, pasty in consistency, analastic? Does it lack crepitance? The parenchyma is now further examined. Does the parenchyma show a consistent uniform appearance, or is it interrupted by a lace-like or punched-out appearance as seen in emphysema? Is the normal color present? Is brownish-orange discoloration present? Needless to say, any lesion should be sectioned for study.

In many autopsies one lung will be surgically absent, having been removed for tumour or, indeed, other conditions. A lobectomy may have been performed. In all such cases the lines of resection should be carefully studied for recurrence of disease. In our laboratory, a section from each pulmonary lobe is routinely taken. In tumour cases a section of carina and several bronchial sections are taken.

The Thymus

Removal of the thymus, where it is found to be present, has already been described. Anatomically, the thymus is divided by a longitudinal fissure which separates the gland into a large right lobe and a smaller left lobe. Persistence of the thymus into adult life may be seen in various diseases, among which chronic intravenous narcotism is but one. The size and weight of the organ should be carefully described with sections taken so as to thoroughly sample the persistent organ.

The Heart

The heart, having already been removed, may now be dissected. It will be remembered that prior to evisceration the vena cavae and pulmonary arteries were opened *in situ*.

Our method of dissection of the heart begins with a separation of the aorta from pulmonary arteries after having ascertained closure of the ductus arteriosus. This separation is obtained by a blunt dissection of the connective tissue remnants of the pericardium which join them. Having separated these two structures, the point of origin of the left coronary artery is located. We prefer to cross cut the artery with a scalpel at millimeter intervals and to follow each branch individually after its bifurcation. Identical dissection of the right coronary artery is performed, having located it at its origin on the right side of the aorta.

It will be remembered that the left coronary artery bifurcates shortly after its origin into the anterior descending, which descends anteriorly along the ventral portion of the interventricular septum to anastomose with the posterior descending which descends posteriorly along the septum. The left circumflex branch of the left coronary passes posterorlaterally to anastomose with the right coronary, thus forming the posterior descending branch. The right coronary bifurcates at the margin of the right ventricle to descend along the margin. After dissection the coronary arteries should be described as to origin, course, relationships, and the presence of atherosclerotic change. Are hemorrhages, acretion or thrombosis present? What degree of atherosclerotic narrowing is present at its best and worst points? Which artery is dominant? The cardiac veins correspond roughly to the arteries and mouth in the coronary sinus which empties into the right ventricle along its posterior surface.

The epicardium is now examined. The approximate quantity of fat, its distribution, and color are noted. Is it yellow and abundant, or is it grey, transparent, gelatinous, and scant?

It should be noted at this point that the heart is opened and examined along the direction of the flow of blood. The incision used to open the vena cava is now extended across the superior surface of the atrium so as to enter and lay bare the right atrial appendage. The atrium is inspected from within. Is the atrial chamber normal in size, or is it dilated? The fossa ovalis is inspected and probed. If a defect is visible, it is described. Probe patency is noted in 25 percent of the autopsies and is without clinical significance. The coronary sinus is inspected, as are the pectinate muscles. Is the endocardium transparent or thickened?

Two fingers are now employed to probe the tricuspid valve. The valve will usually just admit the tips of both fingers. A knife is placed in the atrium through the valve and into the ventricle; its cutting edge is positioned against the margin, and its point exits slightly to the right of the apex. The ventricular chamber should be opened with one cut. The anterior wall of the right ventricle is reflected to the left. This bares the chamber and tricuspid valve. Postmortem clot should be removed and the ventricle washed with a gentle stream of cool water. The valve leaf circumference should now be measured. The valve leaflets are three in number. Are they thin, delicate, and pliable, or are they thick, rigid, and immobile? Are verucca present? Is abnormality noted? The chordae tendineae are examined. Are they thin, or are they thickened and fused? The papillary muscles and trabeculae carneae are examined. What is the character of the endocardium and myocardium? Continuing the dissection in the direction of the flow of blood, the knife edge is now placed with its cutting edge against the septum and through the pulmonary artery. The blade is now turned ninety degrees, and the ventricular wall and pulmonary artery are opened. Again postmortem clot is removed and the ventricle is washed. The pulmonic leaflets are examined, applying the previously stated criteria. The pulmonary outflow tract is examnied. Is it hypertrophied? The pulmonary valve circumference is measured. Again the endocardia and myocardia are examined. The ventricular myocardial thickness is measured 1 cm below the tricuspid valve.

The left atrium is now opened along its superior surface in such a manner as to open the left atrial appendage. Again the endocardia and myocardia are examined. The mitral valve is probed, as was the tricuspid. The knife blade is placed through the atrium and mitral valve and is passed into the ventricle. Its cutting edge is directed against the left cardiac margin, exiting the apex. The ventricle is again opened with one cut. It is washed, clot is removed, and the valve is examined with the same criteria as previously employed. The valve leaft circumference is measured. The knife blade is now placed with its cutting edge against the septum and through the aorta. The cutting edge is rotated ninety degrees and opened with a single cut. The ventricle is washed and clot removed. The aortic valve leaflets are examined, as are the aortic root and coronary ostia. The annulus is palpated. Is it rigid and calcified? The thickness of the ventricular wall is measured 1 cm below the mitral valve. Again, chordae tendineae, papillary muscle, and trabeculae carneae are evaluated.

The septum is now placed against a flat surface and cut along its entire length. The myocardium is evaluated as to the presence of arteries, fibrosis, infarct, or any other abnormality. The anterior wall of the left ventricle is sectioned, as was the septum. Prior to taking section the heart is weighed.

Routine sections are taken in this laboratory through the posterior mitral block, posterior superior interventricular septum and left atrial appendage, as well as through any area of pathology.

Gastrointestinal Tract

The esophagus, duodenum, and stomach, having been removed in continuity with the gallbladder, the common bile duct, and the pancreas are conveniently examined together.

Esophagus

The esophagus is opened along the posterior surface with the distal end of the incision at the greater curvature of the stomach. The incision is then continued along the greater curvature through to the duodenum.

Inspection of the esophagus should include observation of any evidence of tumor or ulceration, whether it be idiopathic or produced by the passage of a nasogastric tube. Should there be a tumor mass seen, it is important to know as far as possible whether the mass is confined to the esophagus or whether it might be directly infiltrating from an adjacent bronchial lesion. The technique for examination of esophageal varices will be discussed below.

Stomach

The stomach is opened along the greater curvature, allowing the open specimen to lie flat. Again, inspection for ulcers or tumor masses is made. The duodenum is opened along the antero-inferior surface and inspected for the presence of ulceration or tumor. If an ulceration is present, it must be determined whether it has penetrated into the pancreas or perforated into the peritoneal space.

When the stomach has been subjected to surgical resection, further observations are necessary. Is the suture line intact, or are these defects or marginal ulcerations? In the case of a gastroduodenostomy, is the duodenal mucosa intact? In the case of a gastrojejunostomy is the blind duodenal stump intact?

Biliary Tree

The inspection of the biliary tree may then be pursued in one of two ways. If the ampulla of Vater is identified, it should be probed for both the common bile duct and the pancreatic duct. If the orifice of the ducts cannot be determined from the duodenal aspect, the alternative method is to follow the ducts from their origin into the duodenum. In this case the gallbladder is incised. Its contents are searched for the presence of calculi. The thickness of the wall is noted. The cystic duct is then opened into the common bile duct. The hepatic ducts are then opened and the common bile duct is opened to its entrance to the duodenum. The presence of calculi are to be noted in any of these ducts.

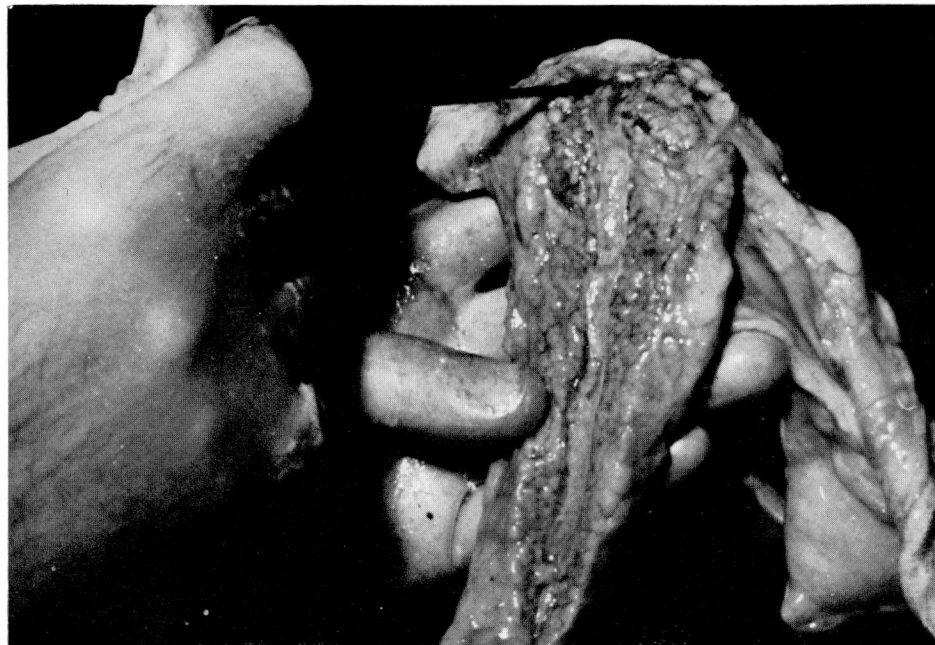

Figure 33

Figures 33 and 34 demonstrate the dissected upper gastrointestinal block. Note dissection of gall bladder and pancreatic duct.

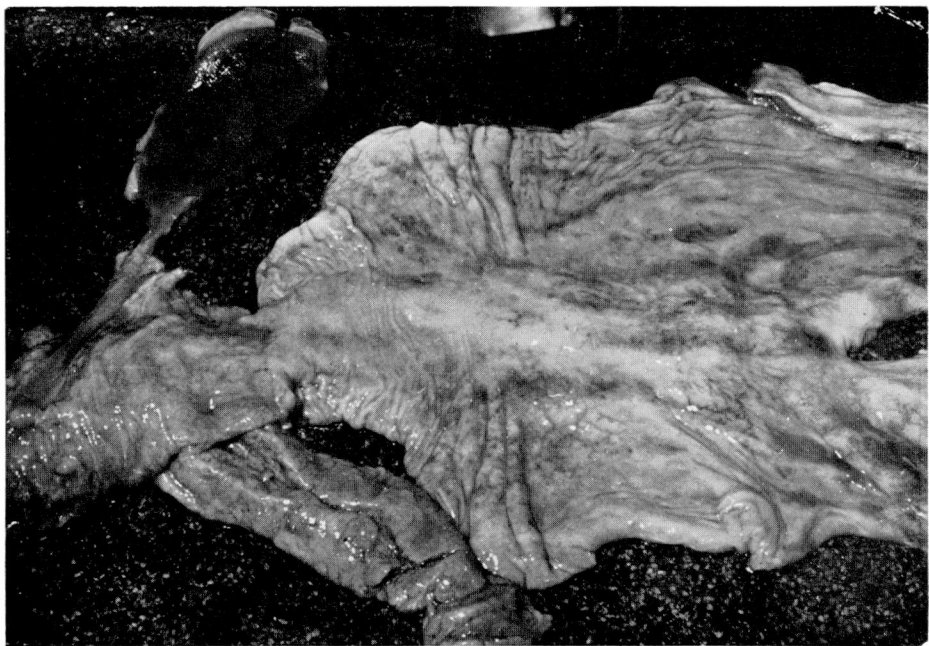

Figure 34

Pancreas

The pancreas is now inspected by means of multiple transverse sections from the tail to the head. Because adenomata of the pancreas may be very small and yet functional, the transverse sections should be no more than 2 to 3 mm apart. The main pancreatic duct (duct of Wirsung) should then be opened into the duodenum. The cut surface of the pancreas should be carefully inspected for the presence of small tumor nodules, cysts, and the presence or absence of fat.

Liver and Spleen

The liver is separated from the diaphragm and lesser omentum by sharp dissection. The external surface is examined for capsular fibrosis and nodularity. Then multiple transverse incisions are made from the anterior to the posterior surface. The sections are examined for nodularity, fibrosis, and the presence of tumors or abscesses. The spleen is sectioned as was the liver.

Esophageal Varices

In searching for esophageal varices several techniques are used. The one most commonly

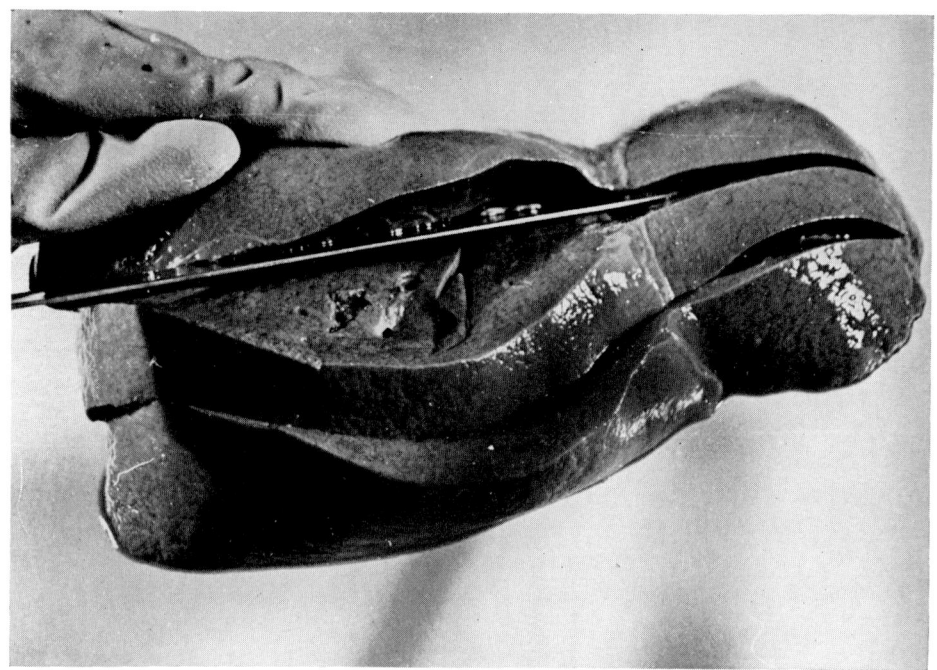

Figure 35

Figures 35 and 36 show the dissection of the liver.

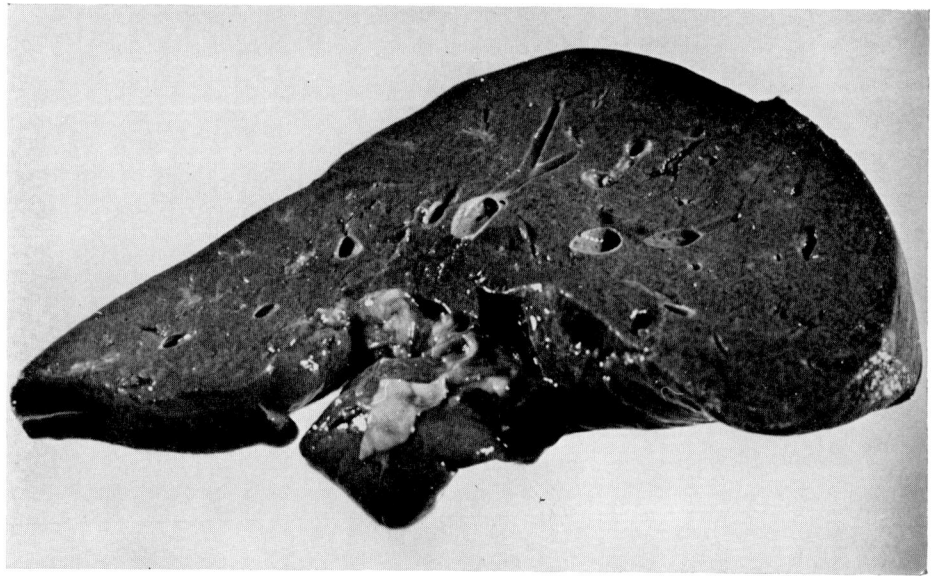

Figure 36

used at this institution is to ligate the superior end of the esophagus, passing a ligature down through the stomach to the duodenal cuff and then by traction on this ligature inverting the entire esophagus and stomach. This prevents, to some extent, the collapse of the distended veins since they are not incised. The esophagus is then examined for the presence of varices. One alternative method sometimes employed is to incise the esophagus on the external sur-

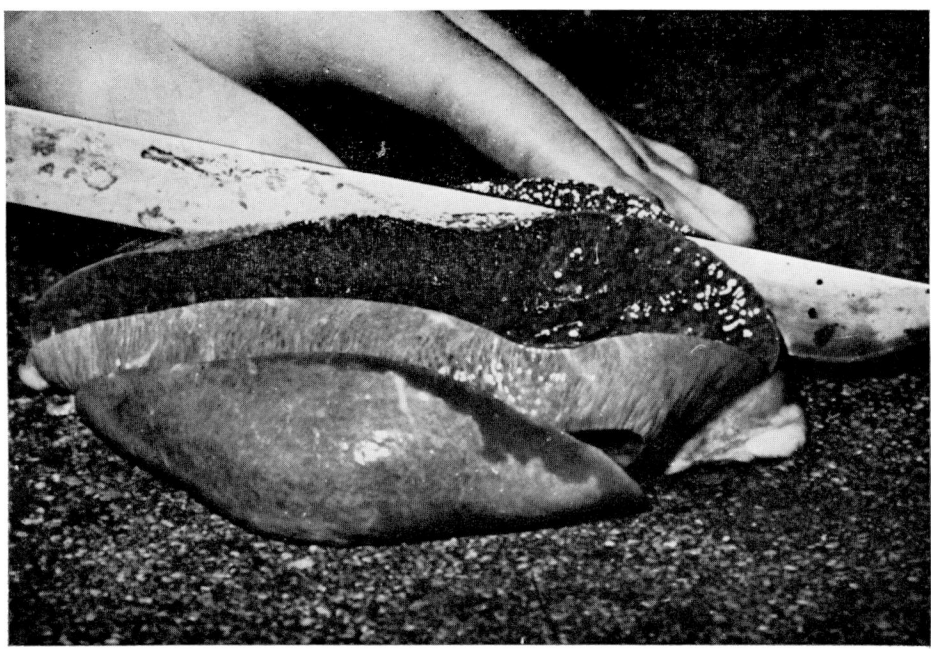

Figure 37

Figures 37 and 38 demonstrate the dissection of the spleen.

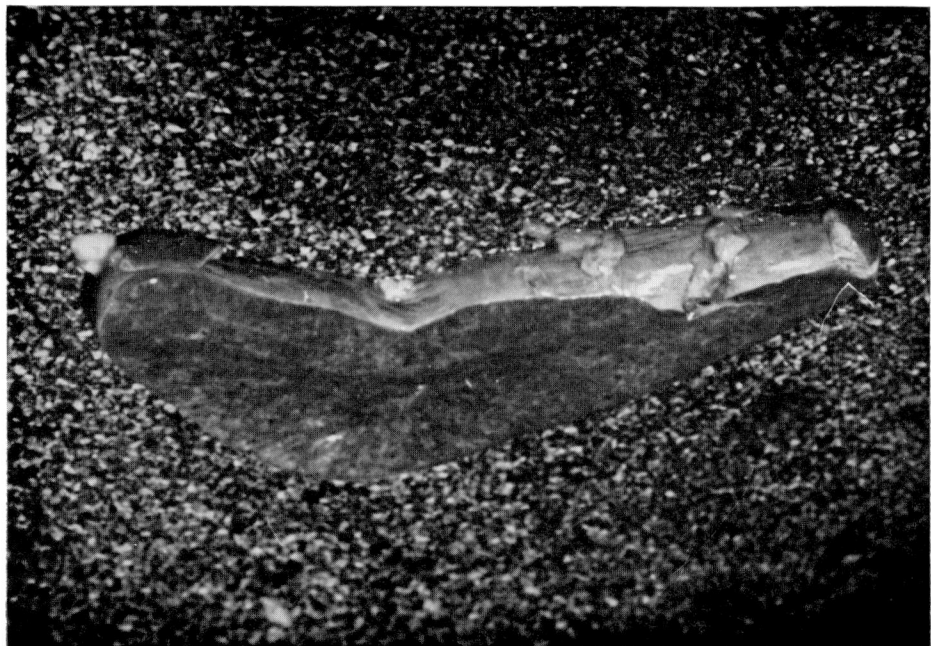

Figure 38

face and to strip the esophageal musculature away from the submucosa where the varices are located.

Small Intestine

The small intestine is examined by enterotome along the antimesenteric border with light traction on the intestine allowing the weight of the enterotome to effect the incisions. The mucosal surfaces are washed with a gentle stream of water and inspected for polyps, ulcers, or other abnormalities. The small intestine is inspected for the presence of diverticula which occur on the mesenteric border, with the exception of Meckel's diverticulum which occurs on the antimesenteric border approximately 70 to 100 cm proximal to the ileocecal valve, representing a remnant of the omphalomesenteric duct. Unlike the smaller diverticula seen on the mesenteric aspect of the intestine which have no muscular wall, Meckel's diverticulum has a well-developed muscularis and often resembles a branching of the small intestine. If present, several microscopic sections are made because of the high incidence of ectopic glands, especially gastric and pancreatic which may be found, and to detect subsequent ulcerations in the diverticulum and adjacent intestine. One abnormality which bears close inspection is intussusception. In adults this is most often associated with a tumor at the leading edge which should be investigated carefully for the presence of even a small polyp.

If the small intestine appears hemorrhagic or dusky, the mesenteric vessels must be examined as described in the chapter on the vascular system.

Large Intestine and Appendix

The colon is opened with the enterotome and washed. It is inspected for the presence of diverticula, here usually seen on the antimesenteric or lateral borders rather than on the mesenteric border. Tumors or ulcerations are noted. For reasons of photography and presentation at conferences, if a large tumor is encountered it is preferable to cut the colonic wall opposite the tumor when possible. The distal colon is also inspected for the presence of hemorrhoids. If a tumor is found, the adjacent mesentery is searched for lymph nodes to determine the presence of metastases.

The vermiform appendix is inspected by a series of transverse cuts including careful examination of its tip which is a frequent site of occult carcinoid tumors.

Genitourinary Tract

Adrenal Glands

It is convenient to include the examination of the adrenal glands along with the kidneys. Whether removed by the Virchow or Rokitansky techniques, the glands should be examined by multicple transverse incisions searching for the presence of nodularity within the cortex, the relative thickness of the medulla and cortex, and the presence or absence of cortical lipid depletion. The thickness of the medulla is noted, as well as the appearance of the central vein.

Kidneys

The kidneys are inspected for the location of the arteries and veins and their relationship to the ureters, abnormalities of which are noted. Any enlarged lymph nodes at the hilum are sectioned.

The kidneys are "bivalved" by a coronal section starting at the lateral border. The capsule is then stripped, and the surface architecture is examined for the presence of scars, cysts, or tumors. The cut surface is examined for the thickness of the cortex, the prominence of glomeruli, the degree to which the corticomedullary junction is preserved and the presence or absence of tumors. The calyces and renal pelves are examined for evidence of dilatation, inflammation, or the presence of calculi. If any of these be present and the ureters appear normal, sections of the ureteropelvic junction are indicated.

If a tumor is noted, careful attention must be directed to the possibility of invasion of the renal vein branches or the renal capsule.

Ureters

The ureters are opened and examined for the presence of calculi, areas of dilatation, or stricture. The mucosal surface should also be examined for the presence of cysts (ureteritis cystica, or ureteritis glandularis), tumors or plaque-like thickenings such as are seen in malakoplakia.

Urinary Bladder

The urinary bladder is opened by an incision on the anterior surface including the urethra. The mucosal surface is inspected as were the ureters for cysts (cystitis cystica or glandularis) tumor and yellowish plaques which may be seen in malakoplakia. The bladder must also be examined for the presence of hemorrhagic areas often secondary to the passage of an indwelling catheter. The dome of the bladder is inspected for persistence of urachal remnants and tumors which may have arisen in the urachus.

The trigone and urethra are then examined. In men the urethra is opened by an anterior incision extending from the bladder to the inferior limit of dissection, be it prostate or penile urethra. In women the incision is similarly made on the anterior surface throughout the length of the urethra with inspection for tumors or inflammatory lesions, particularly urethral caruncles.

In both sexes the external genitalia are examined for ulcerations and the presence of condylomata accuminata which may be present on either the cutaneous surface of the external genitalia or the perianal area.

Female Genital Tract

The female genital tract is examined by means of a posterior incision including the posterior wall of the vagina, the *cervix uteri*, and the body of the uterus. The mucosal surfaces are inspected for the presence of cysts or tumors. The fallopian tubes are inspected by means of multiple transverse sections, and the ovaries are inspected for the presence of adhesions on the surface, cysts, and tumors. Each cystic area must be evaluated for the presence of hemorrhage, which may indicate the presence of endometriosis (chocolate cysts) or ectopic pregnancies.

Male Genital Tract

The male genital tract is examined as follows: The testes are measured and weighed. They are each incised with a single cut, including the epididymis, and examined for the presence of tumors or abscesses, particularly in the epididymis which is the most common site of tuberculosis in the male genital tract.

The prostate is examined by means of multiple transverse incisions from the posterior surface, with attention to the presence of nodularity and areas of necrosis manifest by small areas of yellowish tissue in the subcapsular area. Should such areas be seen, dissection of the seminal vesicles and local fibroadipose tissue, as well as vertebral and pelvic bones, is necessary searching for metastatic foci.

The seminal vesicles are similarly examined by multiple transverse incisions from the posterior aspect with particular attention to the thickness of the wall of the vesicles.

The urethra (as noted above) is seldom examined. Should there be an indication (such as chronic gonococcal urethritis), it is laid open by either an anterior or a posterior incision.

Chapter 3

THE NERVOUS SYSTEM

DIFFICULTIES encountered in the interpretation and diagnosis of pathologic processes involving the nervous system usually result from a disorderly approach, improper technique, or inadequate sampling of tissues at the autopsy table, and not from lack of special expertise in neuropathology on the part of the pathologist. Consultations regarding difficult problems can always be obtained at a later date, but may be of little value if sufficient clinical information, accurate gross anatomic observations, and properly removed and preserved specimens have not been obtained at the time of autopsy.

The goal to be achieved is the removal, with a minimum of anatomical distortion, of all tissues which will be contributory to the diagnosis, and to accurately record, verbally and photographically, abnormalities in structure which cannot be removed or anatomically preserved. The approach and the techniques to be described are those which we have found to be the most efficient and effective in attaining these ends.

REVIEW OF THE CLINICAL RECORD

The deciphering and interpretation of clinical records can be a most arduous task. Success in this endeavor varies with the quality and clarity of the record as well as with the pathologist's clinical acumen. Nevertheless, a clear understanding of the patient's clinical problem before performing the autopsy is often of critical importance in diseases of the nervous system, since alterations in the routine procedure may be dictated by clinical considerations. Examples of such variations in routine include removal of the sella turcica, the petrous bones, the contents of the orbit, and specific peripheral nerves and skeletal muscles.

Therefore, whenever possible, recorded information should be supplemented by direct communication with the clinicians, particularly neurologists and neurosurgeons who were involved in the care of the patient.

EXTERNAL EXAMINATION

An accurate description of visible and palpable abnormalities should be recorded before any incisions are made. Measurement of the circumference of the head is especially important in infants and children. Occasionally it is a useful piece of information to have, even in adults, when atrophic lesions or dilated ventricles, which may have been present from early life, are unexpectedly encountered.

Surgical incisions, lacerations, contusions, and scars should be recorded either on line drawings or, particularly if medicolegal actions could possibly arise from the case, photographically.

The skull should be palpated for areas of depression and soft tissue or boney masses.

The eyes should be examined for prominence, cataracts, corneal ulcerations, pigmentations, and opacities, which occasionally accompany neurologic diseases. Measurement of pupil size, a common practice at autopsy, is of no particular value in the diagnosis of neurologic disease since neurogenic abnormalities of pupil size do not persist after death. Persistence of unequal pupils after death usually indicates disease of the iris.

The body should be turned for inspection of the spinal axis. Specific abnormalities to be sought here are abnormal curvatures, soft tissue masses, and sinus tract openings. The extremities are inspected particularly for muscular atrophy and contractures.

Observations of neurologic importance are not, of course, confined to the areas or abnormalities just specified. Abnormalities noted on any portion of the body surface may be pertinent to the neuropathologic diagnosis.

INSTRUMENTS

One cannot be dogmatic about what specific model or brand of instrument should be used at each step in the brain and cord removal. There are a number of instruments designed to facilitate specific steps in the procedure which, while helpful, are not necessary. Nevertheless, there is a certain amount of basic equipment, in addition to the routine assortment of scalpels, knives, scissors, and forceps, without which the neurologic autopsy cannot be properly executed or will, at least, be tedious and time consuming.

The word "saw," when used in the descriptions to follow, always refers to the electrically powered vibrating saw (Stryker autopsy saw). We have rarely had occasion to use the hand saw, and the electric saw, when properly used, has the advantages of speed, ease of manipulation, and relatively little danger of inadvertently lacerating soft tissues. A large blade that will penetrate to a depth of 1¾ inches is very useful in cutting the vertebral arches for spinal cord removal.

A heavy metal hammer or mallet and the proper assortment of chisels greatly increase the ease with which the boney coverings of the nervous system are removed. The Virchow chisel (head wrench), because of the mechanical advantage it offers, makes removal of even the incompletely cut calvarium a simple matter. A large hatchet-shaped chisel (Councilman's chisel) is necessary to penetrate the depth of the lumbar vertebrae in spinal cord removal.

Bone forceps are very useful at a number of steps in the proceedings. These include opening of the orbit and paranasal sinuses, stripping the dura mater from the base of the skull, and correcting minor errors in the cutting of the vertebrae for spinal cord removal.

THE HEAD AND INTRACRANIAL CONTENTS

Reflection of the Scalp

The incision for reflecting the scalp should be placed in such a location that it will not be visible should the body be displayed in a coffin prior to final disposition. The consideration is obviously of special importance in bald-headed men.

The incision is begun immediately posterior to the root of the auricle on one side and carried to the same point on the opposite side. It passes the midsaggital plane at a point 4 to 5 cm above the external occipital protuberance, varying somewhat with the shape of the skull. The important point is that at least two-thirds of the scalp to be reflected lies anterior to the incision, and when the body is laid in a coffin the incision will be buried in the pillow.

The incision is begun with the sharp edge of the blade toward the skull and in patients with little hair, it may be completed in this manner. However, when abundant scalp hair is present it is generally easier after the initial opening is made to turn the knife so that the cutting edge faces outward and, in short steps, to slide the blade under the scalp and pull outwards, cutting the scalp from its undersurface.

The incision is carried through all layers of the scalp to bone. When this is accomplished, a finger is worked under the anterior edge of the incision and reflection of the anterior scalp flap is initiated. Forward reflection of the scalp is usually easily accomplished by grasping the initially freed-up edge with a moist towel and applying forward traction on it while incising

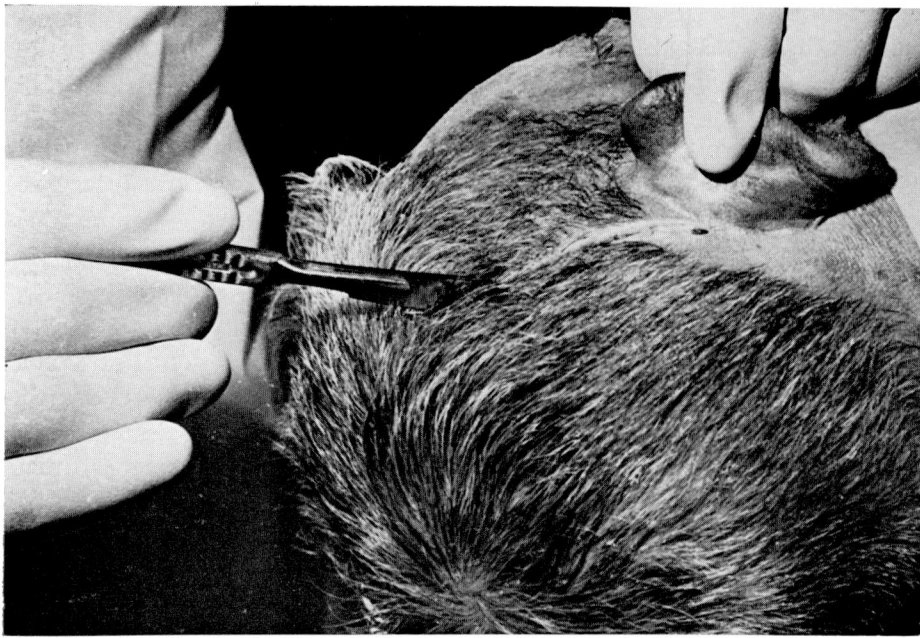

Figure 39. Beginning the scalp incision. Note the proximity of the end of the incision to the root of the auricle.

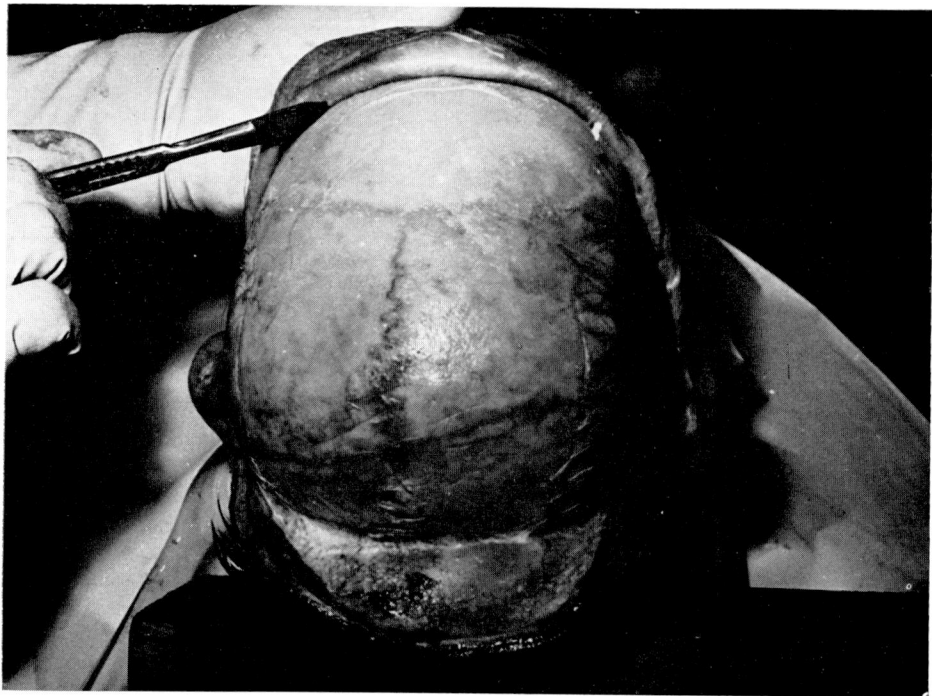

Figure 40. Reflection of the scalp flap.

any adherent bands of periosteum with a scalpel. Difficulty encountered in turning the scalp anteriorly is usually due to failure to extend the incision far enough laterally, or deeply enough, behind the ears. The anterior scalp flap is reflected forward until the calvarium has been exposed to just above the supraorbital ridges.

The posterior edge of the incision is now grasped in a manner similar to the anterior edge

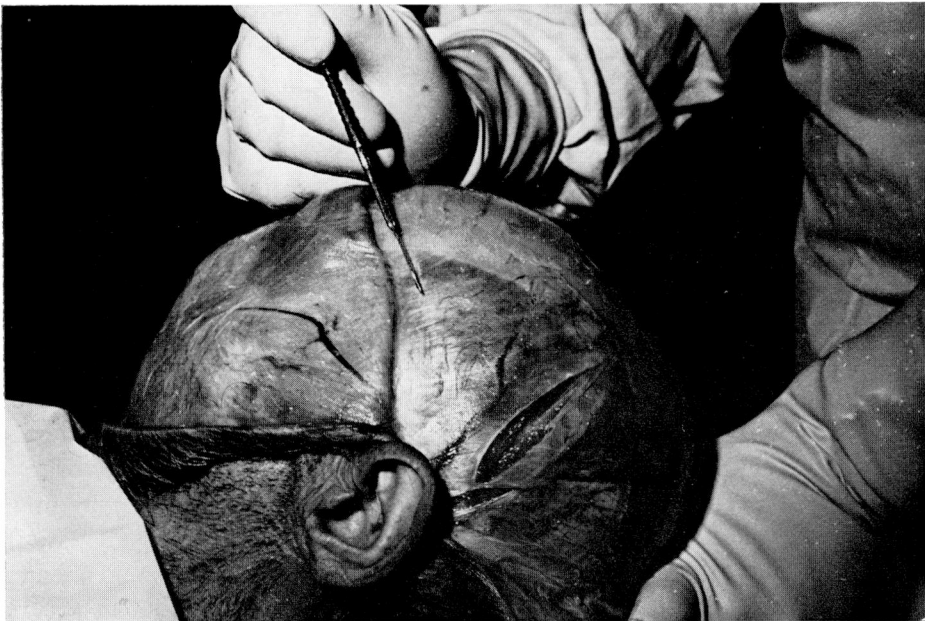

Figure 41. The temporalis muscle exposed.

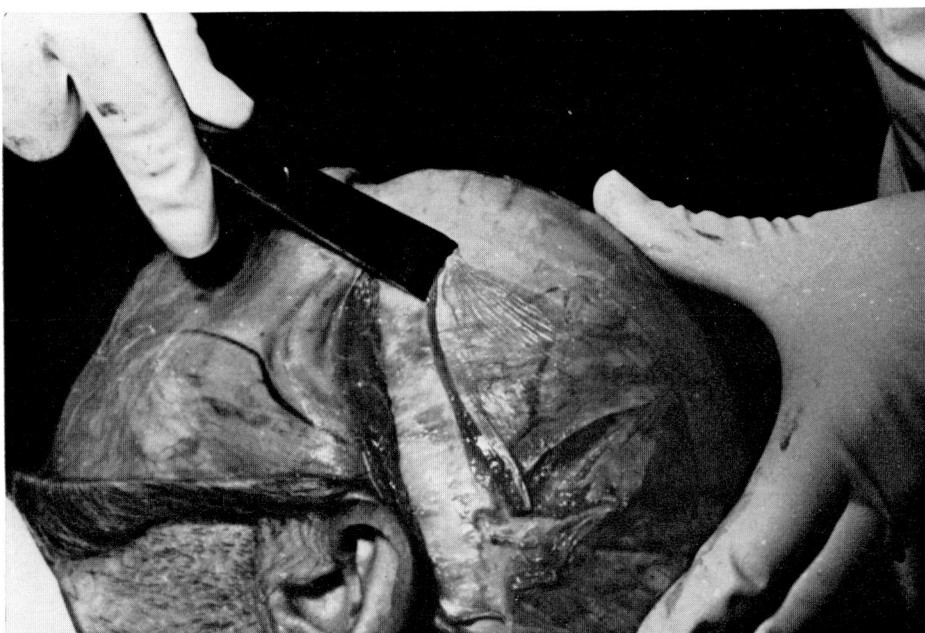

Figure 42. Clearing the temporalis muscle from the temporal bone.

and is reflected posteriorly by combined traction and sharp dissection until the external occipital protuberance is approached. This is generally sufficient to allow the flap to be folded under the neck and out of the way when the calvarium is being cut posteriorly.

The final step in preparing for the removal of the calvarium is to clear the temporalis muscles out of the way, since the vibrating saw is not designed to cut through soft tissue. An incision is made through each muscle in the line of the anticipated saw cut (see next section), and a pathway about 1 cm wide is cleared by scraping the muscle away from the bone with a chisel.

The Calvarium

Anatomical distortions, which are sometimes diagnostically confusing and always aesthically displeasing, arise from two main sources during the removal of the brain. The first is the improper use of the saw while cutting the skull, so that deep lacerations are made into the substance of the brain. The second, more fully explained in the next section, is failure to incise all the attachments holding the brain within the skull, resulting in undue traction upon and tearing of the brain during removal.

The first pitfall may be avoided by employing the following precautions. Except to mark the proposed line of the bone incision with a very superficial groove, the saw should never be run along the skull in a slicing manner, but rather it is pressed directly into the skull with no lateral movement and then withdrawn and moved to the adjacent uncut segment. With experience, one will soon develop the "feel" of having passed through the bone at each point. It is better to make too shallow a cut at some points and retouch them later than to attempt to penetrate the bone completely at all points the first time around. It is very helpful to have an assistant steady the head while the prosector concentrates on cutting the skull. This is especially so when the head must be turned far to one side while cutting the occipital area. It is when this awkward maneuver is attempted by a lone operator that the deepest brain lacerations are usually inflicted.

The design of the bone incision used in removing the calvarium varies from one institution to another. The pattern described below gives maximal exposure to the intracranial cavity, facilitating the removal of the brain without undue traction, and it allows the calvarium to be replaced securely and without danger of slipping after the scalp flaps are replaced.

The bone incision is begun in the anterior midline just above the glabella. It is carried laterally, first on one side and then on the other, to a point 1 or 2 cm above the root of each auricle. The temporalis muscle should have been previously incised and cleared along this pathway.

A right-angle notch, or step, is then created on each side by first making a shortcut perpendicular to and through the posterior end of the first incision line. Another cut is then made perpendicular to and through the upper end of the second. The last mentioned saw cuts are

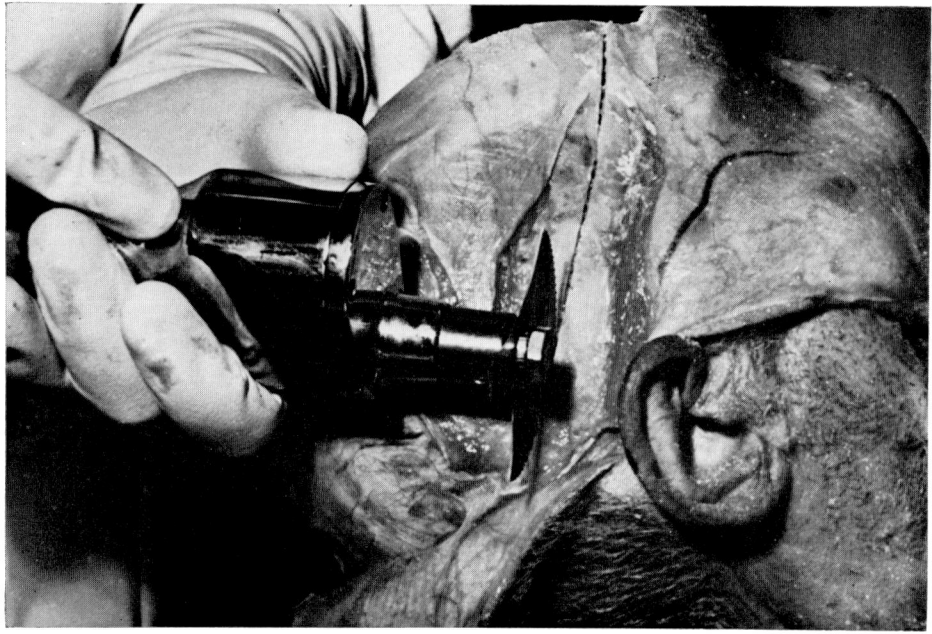

Figure 43. The anterior bone incision.

thus parallel to and about a centimeter above the first incision line, and their ends can now be joined by extending each of them posteriorly to meet in the posterior midline just above the external occipital protuberance. The steps, thus placed in the temporal regions, will ensure a secure fit when the calvarium is replaced.

When the sawing has been completed, the skull cap may still feel firmly attached and immobile and, in fact, if proper caution has

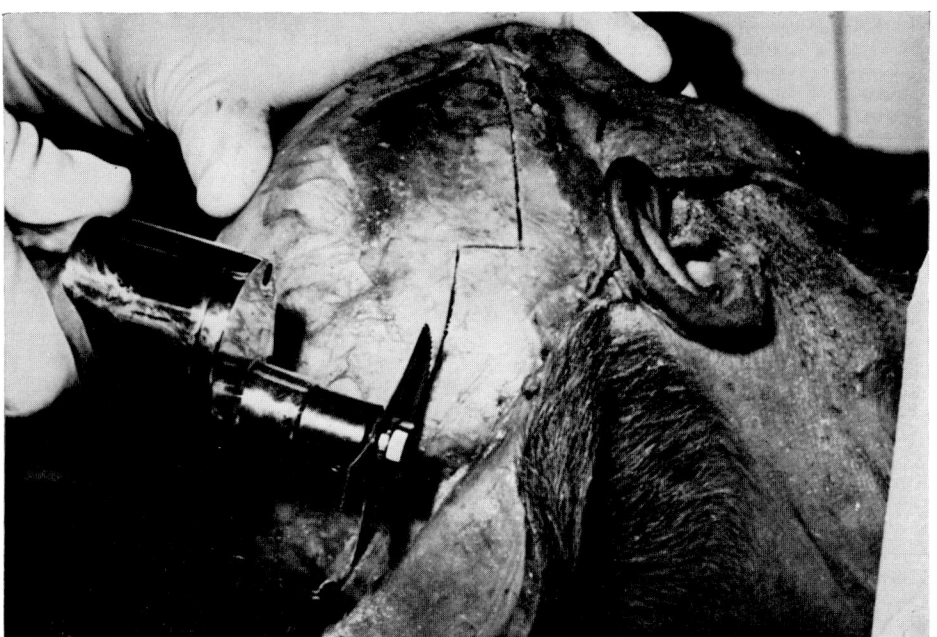

Figure 44. The posterior bone incision. Note the right-angle step in the temporal area.

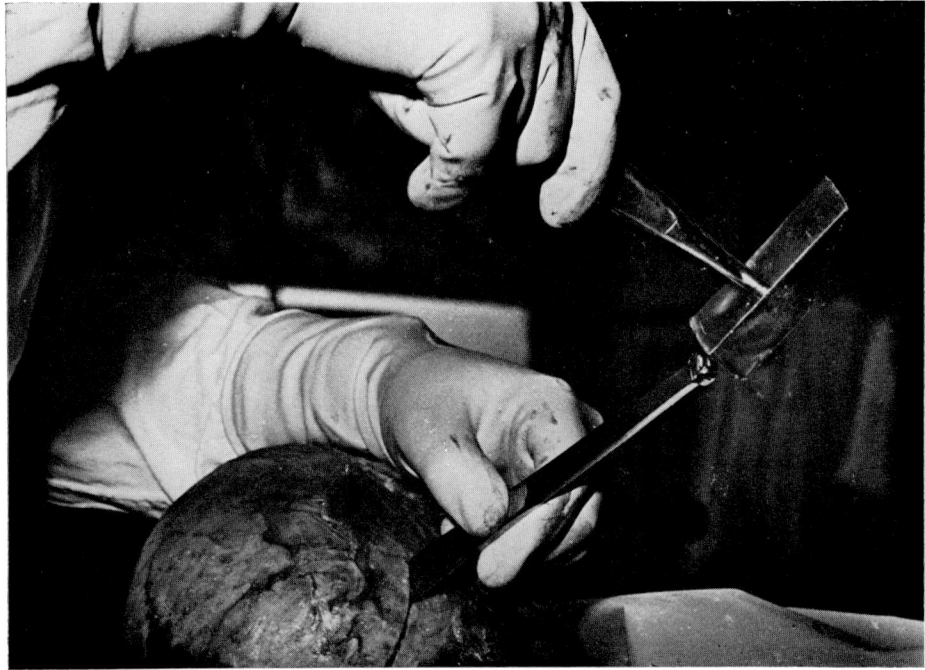

Figure 45. Loosening of the calvarium with chisel and hammer.

been exercised, it usually is still adherent due to thin bridges of bone at various points around its circumference. These boney bridges can generally be fractured by gently tapping around the margins of the saw cut with a chisel and hammer. Once some loosening of the calvarium has been effected, areas of more formidable boney adherence can be identified and the saw cautiously applied to these regions.

After the calvarium has been loosened around its entire circumference, a Virchow chisel is inserted between the bone edges in the anterior

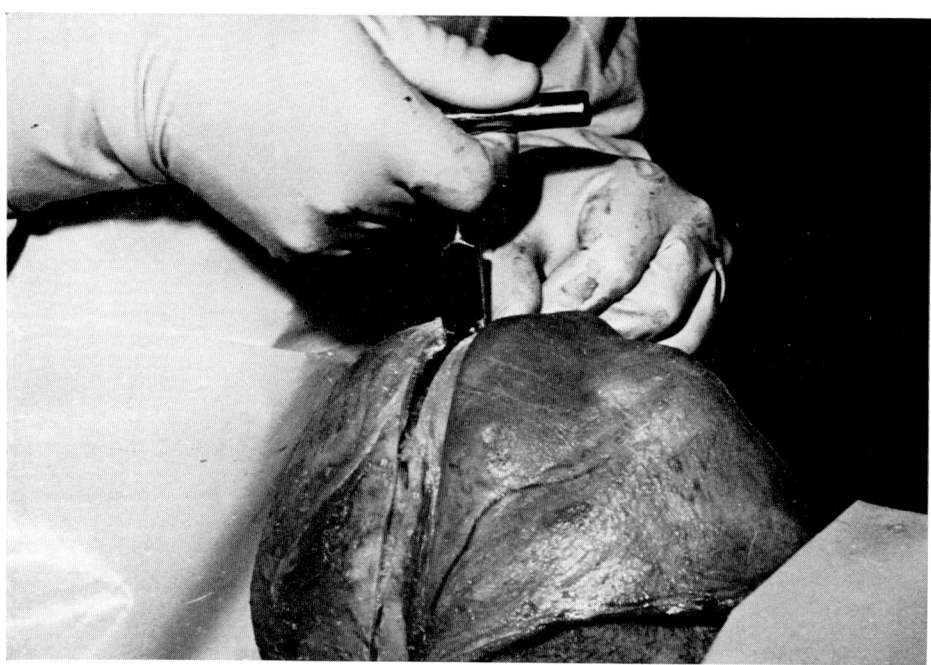
Figure 46. Opening the vault with the Virchow chisel.

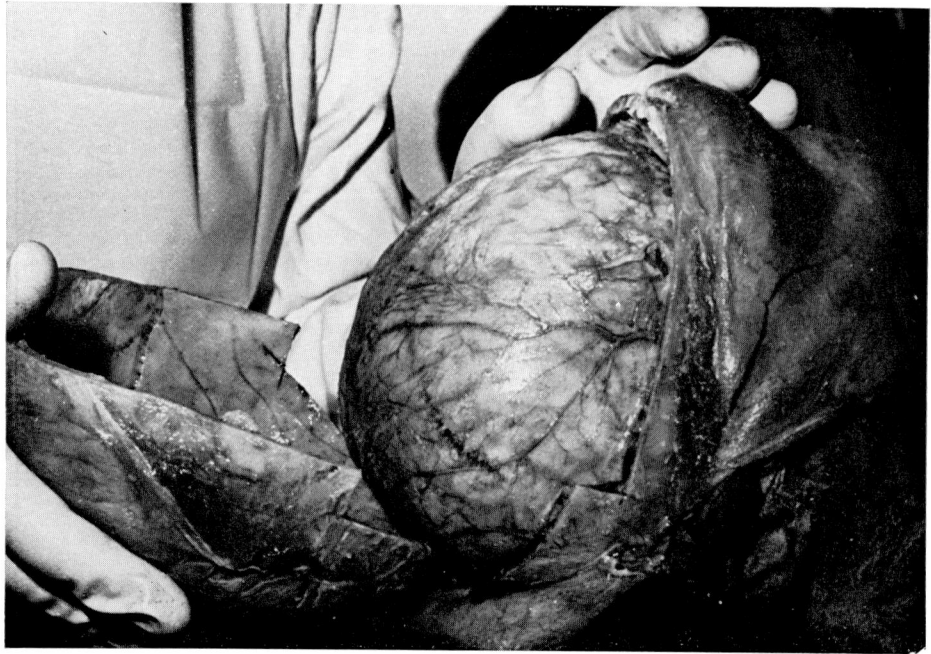
Figure 47. Removal of the calvarium with exposure of the dura.

midline and twisted to separate them. The inner surface of the skull will begin to pull away from the dura. This procedure may be repeated at various points laterally and posteriorly. When the margin of the calvarium has been pulled back far enough, it will become possible to grasp the edge with one hand and apply manual traction. The other hand is inserted into the widening gap between the dura and the inner surface of the skull, gently breaking adhesions between them. The calvarium will come away from the dura with increasing ease and is removed.

Occasionally, especially in young children and in the elderly, or if a considerable portion of the circumference of the dura has been inadvertently incised while cutting the bone, it will be extremely difficult or impossible to begin the separation of skull from the dura. In these instances it is necessary to complete the cutting of the dura with scissors along the line of the separation of the bone edges and remove the calvarium and underlying dura together. One hand is used to grasp and apply traction to the calvarial-dural cap in the same manner as to the calvarium alone under normal circumstances. The other hand is inserted between the undersurface of the dura and the brain and used to gently break arachnoid adhesions and bridging veins as they are encountered.

Before proceeding further with the removal of the brain, the calvarium should be inspected for abnormalities. Suspicious areas may be removed by cutting out squares of bone with the saw. The width of the fragments removed should be no more than about 2 cm to avoid any obvious areas of depression when the scalp flaps are replaced.

The Calvarium in Infancy

The only part of the neurologic autopsy that is basically different in the infant is the opening of the calvarium. The following method is applicable to infants up to 2 or 3 months of age. After this age ossification of the skull has progressed to the point where the usual method of sawing the calvarium is preferable.

The scalp is reflected in the usual manner. An incision is made in the saggital suture line with a scalpel. Then, using scissors, the saggital, metopic, coronal, and lambdoid sutures and underlying dura are cut. The superior saggital sinus and falx cerebri will have been transected at the point where the coronal and lambdoid sutures cross the midline. Having opened the suture lines to their terminations, the two halves of the frontal bone, the parietal bones, and the occipital bone may be spread like the petals of a tulip. Sometimes they must be spread firmly until they crack at their bases in order to keep them apart. The removal of the brain may now proceed in the usual manner.

The Dura

Assuming that the calvarium has been removed in the ordinary manner, the dura over the convexities of the brain, now exposed, is inspected for external abnormalities. An incision is then made using scissors around the entire circumference of the dura, following the outlines of the bone shelf, except at its most posterior pole, the region of the torcular Herophili. The anterior attachment of the falx cerebri to the crista gali is incised and the brain will begin to fall away from the floor of the skull.

Removal of the Brain

During the remainder of the brain removal procedure, one hand should be cupped over the cerebral hemispheres at all times with the brain gently resting on it. This is to prevent the brain from precipitously falling backwards as the attachments to the base of the skull are severed. The free hand is used to gently coax the brain backward from its undersurface and to sever the nerves, vessels, and fibrous attachments of the brain with a scalpel or very sharp scissors as they are encountered.

The first structures to appear when the frontal lobes are lifted back are the olfactory bulbs and tracts. A sharp scalpel blade is worked into the olfactory groove beneath the bulbs, severing the olfactory nerve twigs which pass through the cribiform plate. The optic nerves are then visualized and are sectioned as close to the optic foramina as possible. The internal carotid arteries are sectioned as they pass upward immediately behind and lateral to the optic nerves. Finally, the pituitary stalk is sectioned as it passes through its hiatus in the diaphragm of the sella.

The brain has now been freed of all its attachments in the anterior and middle cranial fossae except for occasional adhesions between the leptomeninges and basal dura which may be lysed by blunt or sharp dissection as required. As the brain is rotated slightly more posteriorly, the third cranial nerves will be seen crossing the tentorial notch and entering

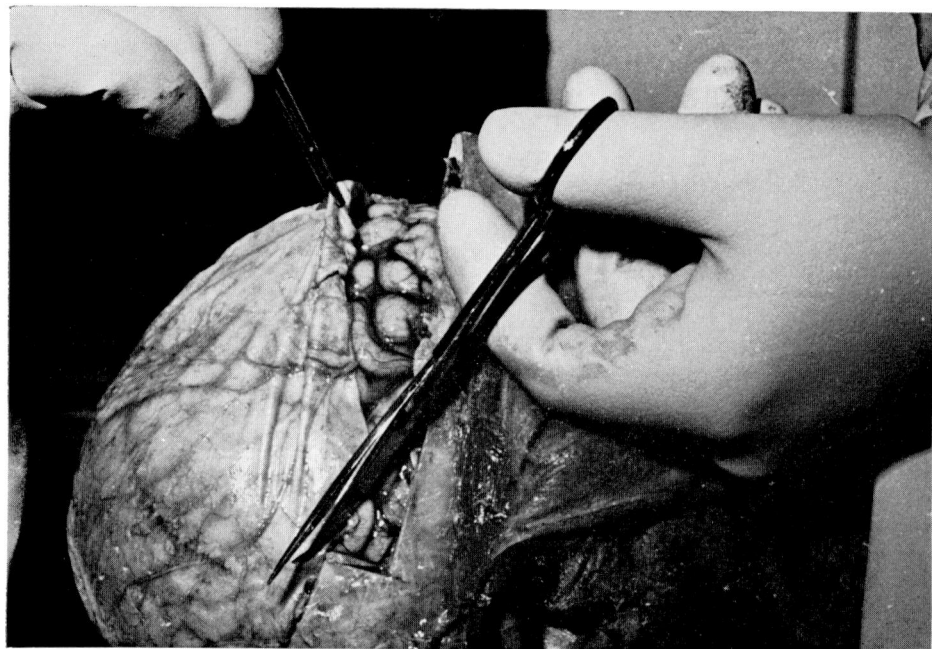
Figure 48. Incising the dura.

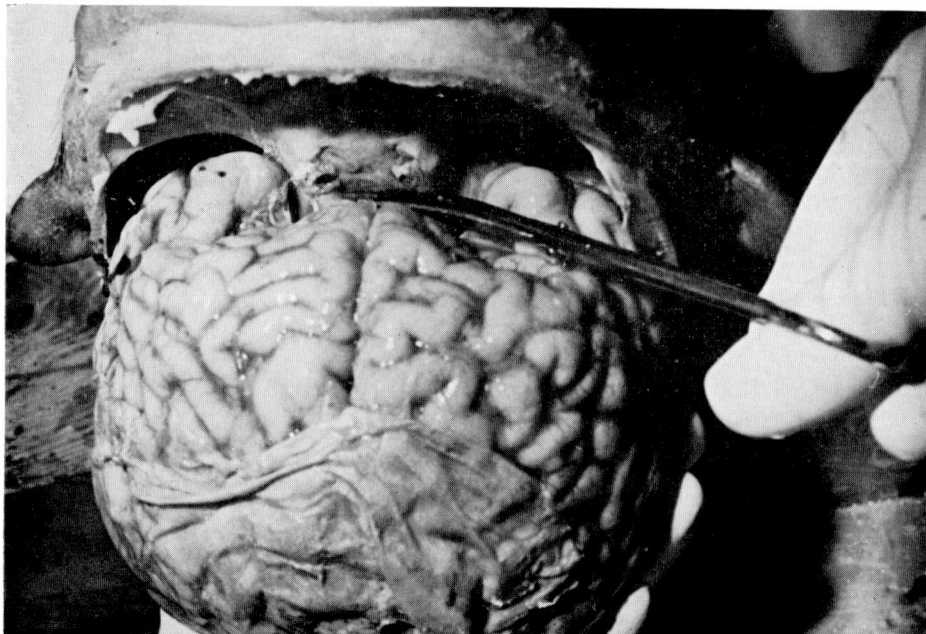
Figure 49. Transection of the optic nerve as it enters the optic foramen.

the posterior wall of the cavernous sinus. They should be severed close to the sinus as soon as they come into view since more than slight traction upon them as the brain is rotated backwards will cause them to be torn from their roots at the base of the midbrain.

The next maneuver, the cutting of the tentorium cerebelli, is one of the most crucial steps in proper brain removal. Failure to completely incise the anterolateral attachment of the ten-

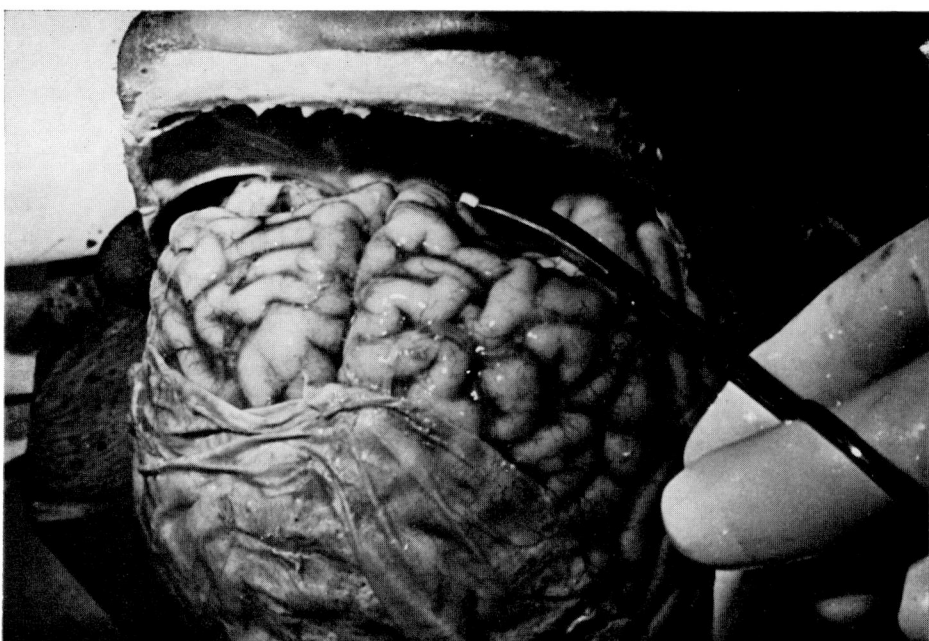

Figure 50. Transection of the pituitary stalk. Note the cut ends of the optic nerves and the internal carotid arteries.

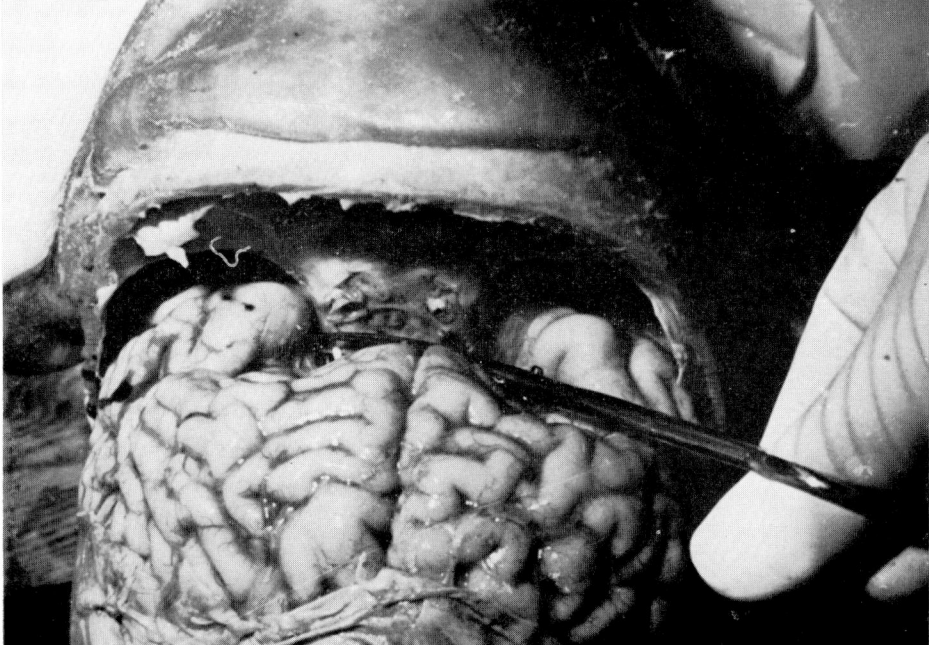

Figure 51. Sectioning the left oculomotor nerve as it enters the posterior wall of the cavernous sinus.

torium to the petrous ridge and the lateral and posterior attachment to the lateral sinus will cause undue traction to be placed upon the brain stem as the brain is rotated far posteriorly while attempting to section the lower cranial nerves. This will result in tearing, or even avulsion, of the cerebral peduncles from either the pons or diencephalon. This can be a sufficiently serious distortion to impair diagnostic studies.

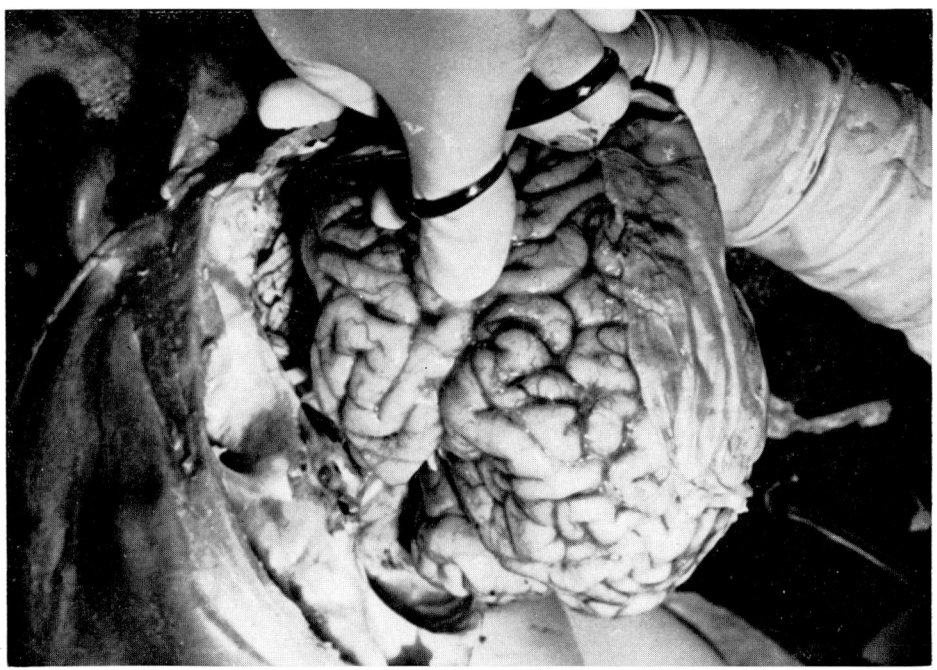

Figure 52. Cutting the tentorium cerebelli. Note that the incision is carried around the posterolateral attachment of the tentorium to the lateral sinus.

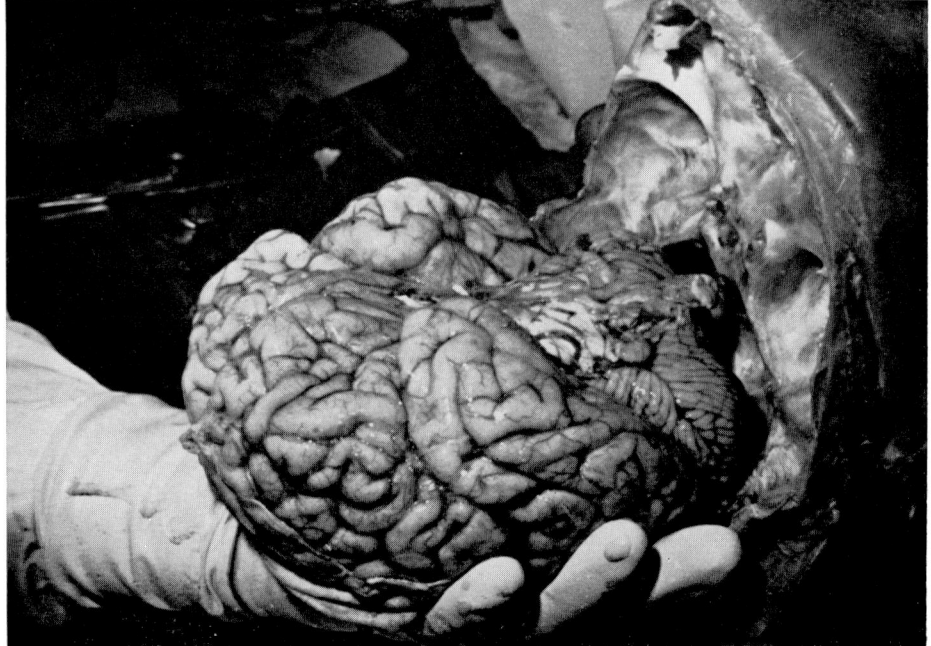

Figure 53. The brain is removed after transecting the upper cervical cord.

The tentorium is most conveniently cut with a long, sharp, slightly curved pair of scissors. Starting at the attachment of the free edge of the tenotrium to the petrous tip, the incision is carried out laterally along the petrous ridge. At its lateral extremity, the corner is turned and the incision is continued along the lateroposterior attachment of the tentorium to the lateral sinus. It is usually possible, without putting undue stress upon the brain, to incise the tentorium almost to the posterior midline at the torcular Herophili. This remaining attachment will be cut later as the final step in actually separating the brain from the skull.

When the tentorium has been cut, cranial nerves IV to XII are easily identified and transected in succession. Often the IVth and Vth nerves will have been inadvertently transected while cutting the tentorium, since they pass very close to its undersurface as they pass forward into the middle fossa. The VIth nerves are extremely thin as they pass upward toward their dural foramina in the upper clivus, and they can be torn with the slightest tension. Therefore they should be sectioned as soon as it is possible to identify them as the brain is rotated back. The remaining cranial nerves are identified in order and transected at their foramina of exit.

The vertebral arteries which pierce the dura and enter the cervical subarachnoid space on either side of the first cervical segment, are now cut with a long pair of scissors. Direct visualization of the arteries usually requires direct light from a flashlight or floor lamp. In the absence of these luxuries, they may be cut "blindly," along with the upper cervical roots and dentate ligaments by snipping along each side of the vertebral canal. As long as the boney wall of the canal is hugged, no damage will be done to the cervical spinal cord.

The mobilization of the brain is now completed by sectioning the spinal cord between the second and third cervical segments with a scalpel. When this is completed the brain should roll back into the supporting hand. The free hand may be slipped around the undersurface of the cerebellum to free any arachnoid adhesions and gently deliver the brain into the supporting hand.

The brain is now completely free of its attachment to the skull, except at the posterior margin of the tentorium cerebelli which is now viewed from its undersurface. When this is sectioned, the delivery of the specimen is completed.

Fixation of the Brain

As a general rule, the brain should be handled as little and as gently as possible at the autopsy table. It may be weighed and the external surfaces are inspected for gross abnormalities. The brain sould then be suspended in formalin solution and fixed for 1 to 2 weeks prior to definitive examination.

The container used for fixation should be large enough to contain 15 to 20 liters of formalin solution, and to allow the brain to hang freely without contact with the walls. In this laboratory, 20% formalin in 1% acetic acid is used for initial fixation because the results of certain staining methods have been empirically found to be superior when this solution is used.

Suspension of the brain is accomplished by passing a piece of heavy twine between the basilar artery and the base of the pons. The brain is then lifted into the bucket and allowed to submerge to a depth at which only slight tension is exerted in the basilar artery as it is held by the string. The ends of the string are then fastened to the rim of the container, 180 degrees apart, by tying them to the handle attachments. The brain is left suspended in formalin for 10 to 14 days before cutting.

Exceptions to the general rule of not disturbing the specimen occasionally arise. In the case of massive subarchnoid hemorrhage due to suspected aneurysm, it is usually preferable to photograph the specimen in the fresh state and then, using forceps and a gentle stream of cold water, wash away as much blood as possible and search for the aneurysm. It is extremely difficult to locate and demonstrate an aneurysm in a solid mass of fixed blood.

It is only under the most extraordinary circumstances that the brain should be cut before it is thoroughly fixed. These circumstances are almost exclusively confined to a medical examiner or coroner's practice where the prompt expedition of justice may demand immediate confirmation or exclusion of a lethal intracerebral lesion. Pathoanatomical studies generally cannot be carried out as well on unfixed material or on brain slices fixed after cutting. If a "yes or no" answer regarding the presence of a lethal intracerebral lesion is required at the time of autopsy, a single cornal section through the cerebrum at a level immediately posterior to the mammillary bodies may be made. If this is unrevealing, a transverse section through the brain stem and cerebellum at the midpontine level may be made. It is almost inconceivable that the presence, location, and, usually, the nature of a lethal macroscopic intracerebral lesion will not be revealed by these two sections when combined with information derived from the external examination of the brain, such as hippocampal herniation, areas of swelling, softenings, and subarachnoid blood. After the cut has been made and the desired information obtained, the two halves of the brain should be placed at the bottom of a container, cut surfaces down, in the usual volume of 20% formalin.

The Base of the Skull, Dural Sinuses, and Pituitary Gland

The remainder of the "routine" portion of the intracranial autopsy may now be completed by inspecting the base of the skull for fractures or other lesions. Inspection of suspicious areas is facilitated by stripping the basal dura from the floor of the skull. This is accomplished by grasping the edge of dura, previously incised during brain removal, with a bone forceps, and pulling it away from the base. If a lesion of the fifth cranial nerve is suspected, the gasserian ganglion, exposed in the manner, is removed from its bed on the medial third of the petrous ridge, labeled appropriately, and placed in formalin.

Even before the dura of the base of the skull is stripped, the dural sinuses, especially the lateral and sigmoid sinuses, should be opened along their lengths in search of obstructions. This is most easily accomplished by beginning

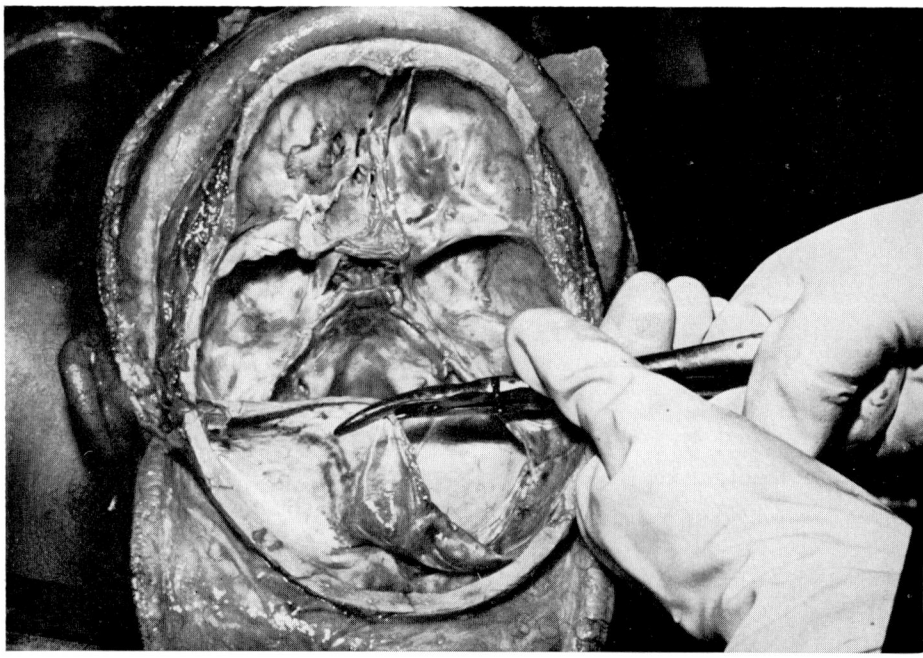

Figure 54. Stripping the dura from the floor of the skull with bone forceps.

at the torcular Herophili and opening each side in turn, longitudinally, with a pair of scissors. Each sinus is traced from the torcular to the beginning of the jugular vein in the jugular foramen. The right sinus is generally larger than the left.

The pituitary gland may be removed in the following manner. The edge of a chisel is placed upon the upper anterior surface of the dorsum sellae, almost perpendicular to the plane of the dorsum. A sharp blow is applied to the chisel with a mallet, fracturing the dorsum sellae off and opening the sella. The diaphragm of the sella can now be easily grasped with a forceps and cut around its circumference with a small pair of scissors. With slight traction on the diaphragm the pituitary gland is then plucked out.

The Sella Turcica and Clivus

The removal of the sella turcica, parasellar tissue, and clivus (basisphenoid and basioccipital bones) in a block is indicated in a variety of conditions. Included among these many conditions are intrasellar or spenoid sinus tumors, intracavernous carotid occlusions and aneurysms, carotid-cavernous fistulas, tumors of the clivus such as chordomas, cavernous sinus infections and thromboses, and intracavernous lesions of the nerves to the extraocular muscles.

The removal of this block is not at all difficult. Four deep cuts are made with the vibrating saw. In contrast to the delicacy which is employed while cutting the calvarium, in this dissection the saw may be used with force and may penetrate up to the hilt without damaging important structures. The first incision is made anterior to the tubercum sellae and perpendicular to the floor of the anterior fossa. A second cut, parallel to the first, is placed in the clivus, usually in its middle to upper third unless the lower third of the clivus is also required for examination. In executing the second cut the saw blade is not directed perpendicular to the plane of the clivus but rather parallel to the floor of the anterior cranial fossa and therefore perpendicular to the plane of the first cut and at an angle of about 45 degrees to the plane of the clivus. The rectangular bone incision is completed by placing a cut on each side of the sella, lateral to the cavernous sinus and perpendicular to and intersecting the ends of the first two incisions. Loosening of the block is now completed by driving a chisel into the incision lines. This will fracture any remaining boney attachments such as the nasal septum, which may still anchor the block. Once mobilized, the specimen is removed by traction, cutting the soft tissues adherent to its undersurface. The block is placed in formalin for future study.

If the entire length of the optic nerve is also to be studied, it should be removed by unroofing the optic foramen and orbit, as described below, before removing the sella. Otherwise the portion within the foramen will be macerated as the saw cuts across the anterior clinoid process.

The Petrous Bone

The pathologic examination of structures contained within the petrous portion of the temporal bone, especially the middle and inner ear apparatus, is a highly specialized procedure and not a practical undertaking in most pathology laboratories. Nevertheless, if study of these structures is contemplated, the specimen is easily removed in much the same manner as the sella turcica and surrounding structures. Two deep saw cuts are made perpendicular to the petrous ridge. One is placed just medial to the internal auditory meatus. The second is placed parallel to the first and about 3.5 cm posterolateral to it along the petrous ridge. A third cut, intersecting the anterior ends of the first two, is made along the anterior border of the petrous bone with the blade directed almost perpendicular to the floor of the middle fossa. The block is completed by making a fourth cut on the posterior aspect of the petrous bone, within the posterior fossa, about an inch below the crest of the ridge with the blade directed parallel to the plane of the floor of the skull and intersecting the posterior ends of the first two cuts. The block is then loosened with mallet and chisel, and removed.

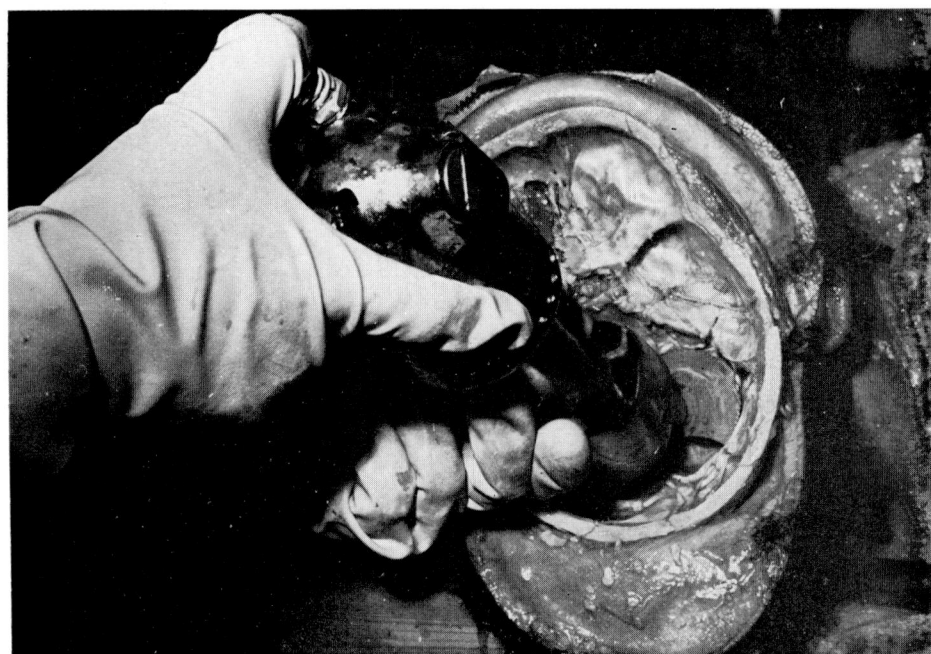

Figure 55. The final saw cut for the removal of the petrous bone containing the inner ear structure.

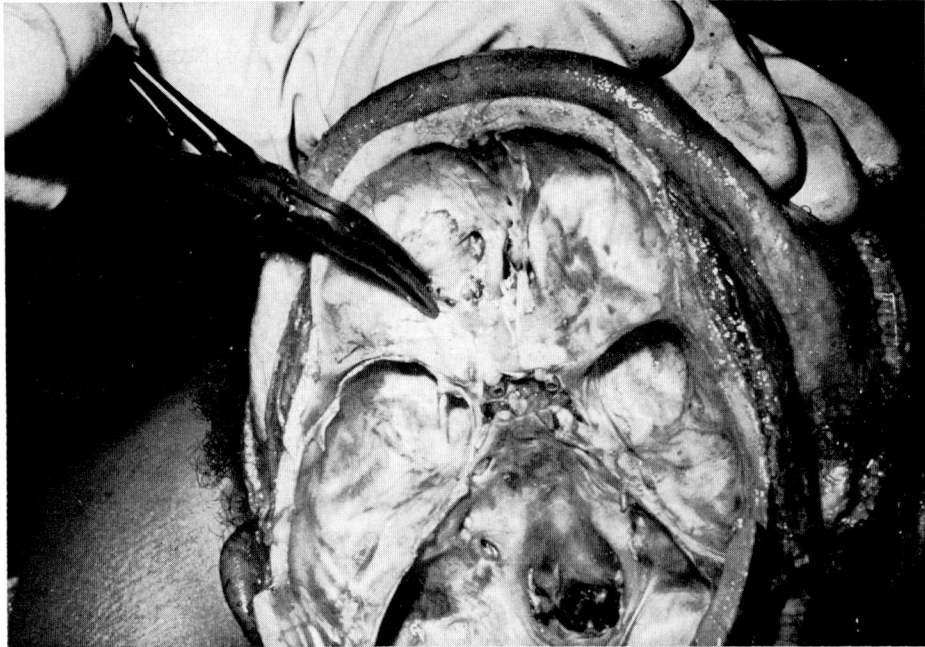

Figure 56. Opening the orbital roof with bone forceps.

The Orbit

Signs and symptoms referable to the eye or other intraorbital structures are frequently encountered in neurologic diseases. Study of the contents of the orbit, therefore, is often a pertinent part of the neuropathologic examination.

Opening of the orbit is easily accomplished by breaking through the thin orbital roof with a chisel and mallet and then biting the bone away in all directions with bone forceps until the orbital contents are completely exposed.

If a specific intraorbital structure such as the

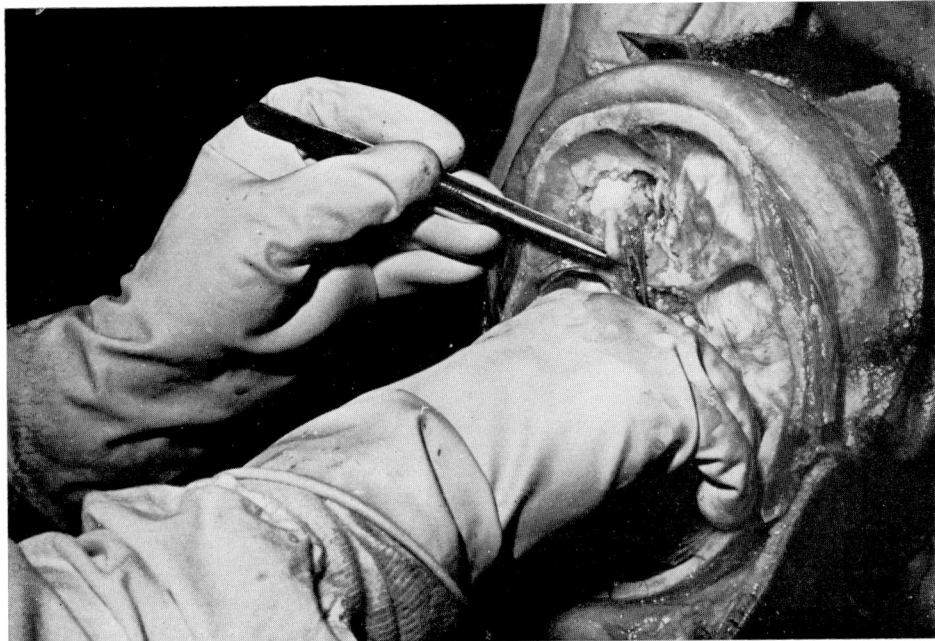

Figure 57. Exposure of the globe and optic nerve.

ciliary ganglion, an extraocular muscle or nerve is being sought, the subsequent dissection must be carried out with great care. The structures which are usually of neuropathologic interest, however, are the retina and optic nerve and the orbital fat, along with the extraocular muscles and nerves which may be dissected away quickly with a small pair of scissors.

The optic nerve is easily identified and traced from the optic foramen to the back of the globe. The orbital fat and extraocular muscles are then cut away from the posterior half of the globe.

At this point one of two procedures may be followed. In situations where special consent is required for removal of an eye and has not been obtained, the posterior half of the globe, which will give an adequate sampling of retina for most purposes, may be removed without violating the restriction. An incision is made with a scalpel across the dorsal surface of the globe at its equator. The incision is completed around the rest of the equator with small sharp scissors. The posterior half of the globe with attached optic nerve is removed. The orbit is then repacked with cotton, muscle, fat, or whatever else is convenient. The external appearance of the eye will remain unaltered.

In situations which permit the total removal of the eye, this is easily accomplished by cutting the muscular and facial attachments of the globe. Care should be taken to avoid lacerating the eyelids. When the removal of the globe is completed, the margins of the eyelids are sewn together from the inside using fine gauge surgical suture material. The orbit is then packed, or a prosthetic globe is inserted in such a manner as to give a normal external contour to the closed lids.

THE SPINAL CORD

A variety of approaches to the removal of the spinal cord have been described. Probably the best approach for a thorough patho-anatomical study of the spinal cord and its relationships, is the removal and fixation of the entire vertebral column as a block. This is achieved by cutting through the sacro-iliac joints, ribs, and atlanto-occipital joints. This procedure, however, besides sounding formidable, requires some artificial restructuring of the body with wood and plaster, and the specimen requires a rather large, special container for fixation. It is, therefore, not easily adapted to most general pathology laboratories.

The posterior approach to the removal of the spinal cord is usually reserved for those uncommon instances in which permission for postmortem examination of the thoraco-abdominal organs has been refused, but for the central nervous system examination has been granted. The body is placed in the prone position with a wooden block under the upper chest. A longitudinal incision is made in the midline from the external occipital protuberance to the sacrum. Muscle must then be cleared from both sides of the vertebral spinous processes and laminae along the length of the spine. The laminae are then cut with a saw on each side of the spinous processes, 1.5 cm from the midline. The remainder of the procedure, including loosening and extraction of the bone and mobilization and removal of the cord, is done in the same manner as in the anterior approach described below. The somewhat greater ease with which the upper few cervical segments of the cord are approached by this method is balanced on the negative side by the lesser accessability of the dorsal root ganglia and distal roots as compared to the anterior approach. Morticians have occasionally voiced objections to the posterior approach on the grounds that incisions on dependent portions of the body tend to leak embalming fluid.

In the usual course of events, the anterior approach to the removal of the spinal cord is adopted. This procedure is carried out in the following manner. After all the pelvic, abdominal, thoracic, and cervical viscera, as well as the brain, have been removed, a wooden block is placed under the back in the upper thoracic area, causing the thoraco-cervical spine to arch slightly dorsally. As much soft tissue as possible is dissected away from the vertebral bodies and pedicles. The insertions of the iliopsoas muscle on the lumbar vertebrae and the prevertebral muscles attached to the cervical spine are the major soft tissue masses to be cleared away. In the course of this dissection the sympathetic chain and ganglia will be found in the retroperitoneal and retropleural spaces lateral to the vertebral bodies, and they may be removed for study.

When the soft tissues have been cleared away, the saw is used to cut through the pedicles on both sides, from the fifth lumbar vertebra below to the highest accessible cervical level above. Generally, it should be possible to cut as high as the fourth, or even the third cervicle pedicles.

The angles at which the pedicles are cut changes at different levels of the spine. In the lumbar spine, the pedicles pass almost directly dorsally from the bodies of the vertebrae. Therefore, in order to transect them, the blade of the saw is directed in a plane parallel to the table top. In the cervical spine, on the other hand, they are directed laterally and therefore transection requires that the plane of the saw blade be perpendicular to the table. Through the thoracic spine, the vertebral configuration gradually shifts from dorsally directed pedicles in the lower portion to more lateral angulation of the pedicles in the upper portion. The plane of the saw, therefore, should be angled somewhat towards the table through most of the thoracic spine, the angulation increasing as the spinal column is ascended. Another aspect of the dissection of the thoracic area which is an occasional source of difficulty is that, unlike in the lumbar and cervical areas, the pedicles are not directly visible or palpable. They are covered by the articular processes of the ribs which pass anterior to them to articulate with the vertebral body. There is a tendency to pass the saw blade anterior to the tip of the rib process. An incision directed in this manner will cut through the body rather than the pedicle of the vertebra, making it necessary to extend the vertebral opening later, creating extra work. To avoid this, each rib articulation should be identified and the saw passed directly through it a few millimeters from its tip rather than anterior to it. If the saw blade is continued inward at the proper angle, the pedicle will be transected.

After the pedicles are transected along the length of the vertebral column, a transverse saw

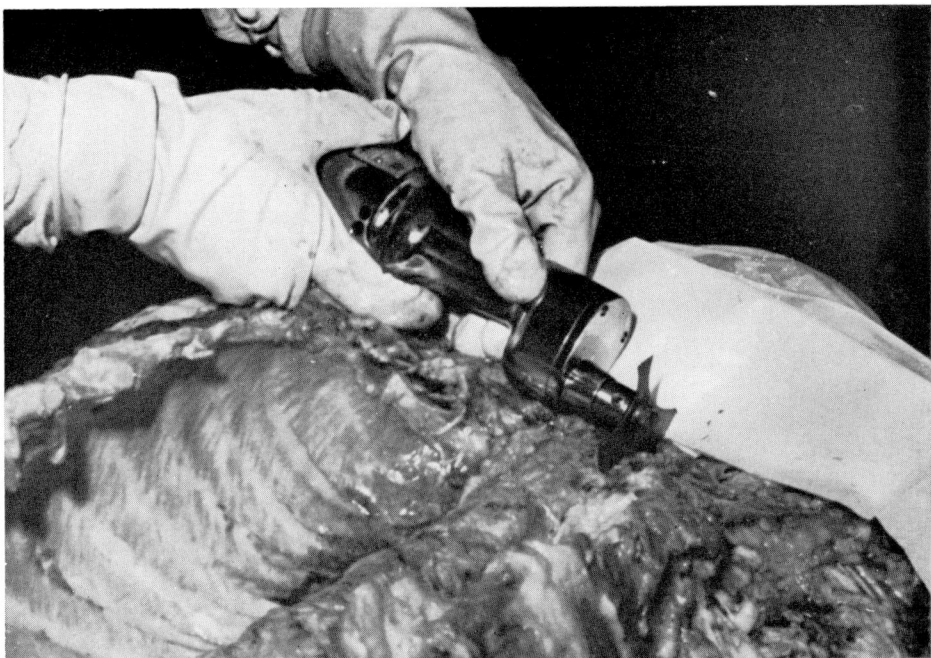

Figure 58. Sectioning the cervical pedicles. Note that the saw blade is directed perpendicular to the tabletop.

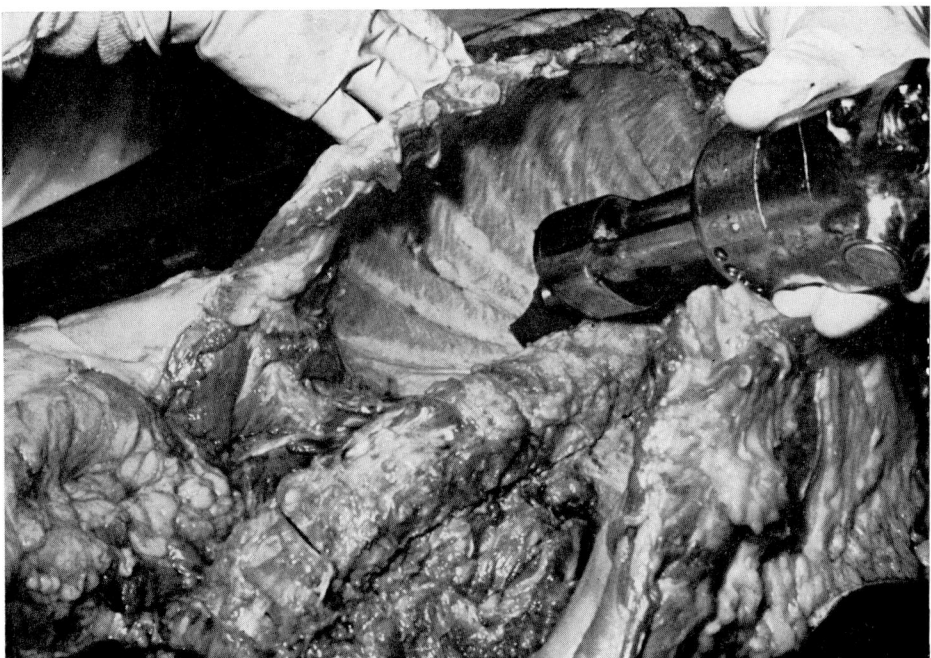

Figure 59. Sectioning the thoracic pedicles. Note that the saw blade is directed at an angle of 45 degrees to the tabletop.

cut is made through the body of the fifth lumbar vertebra. Then a large hatchet chisel is driven into the saw incision line and twisted until the lower end of the column begins to pull loose. Once it is initially mobilized at the lumbar level, and provided the pedicles have been properly cut, it should be possible to manually pull off the entire column of vertebral bodies in one piece, except for the upper three or four cervical segments.

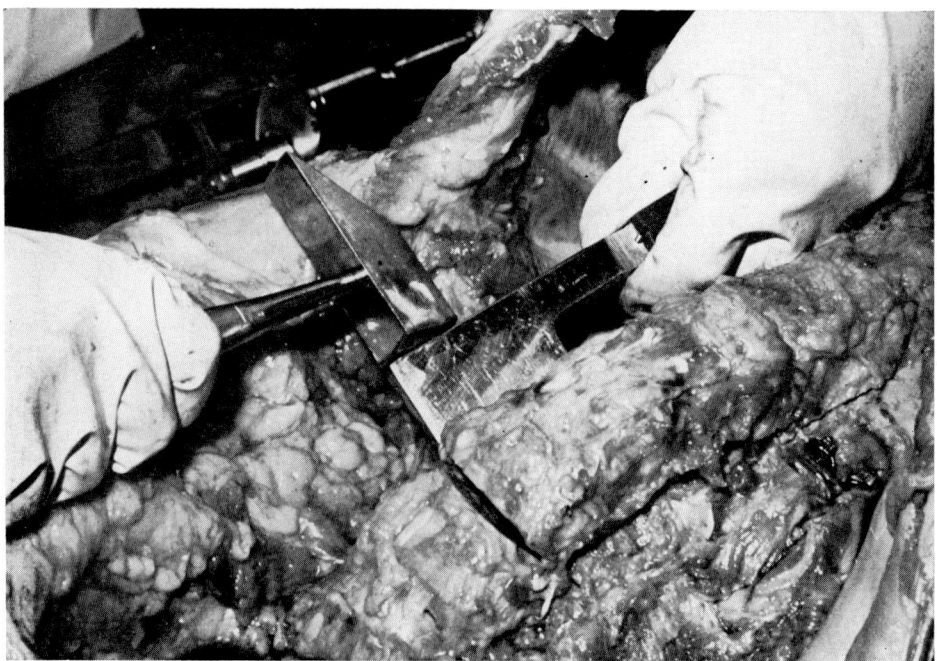

Figure 60. Loosening the lower end of the spinal column with chisel and hammer.

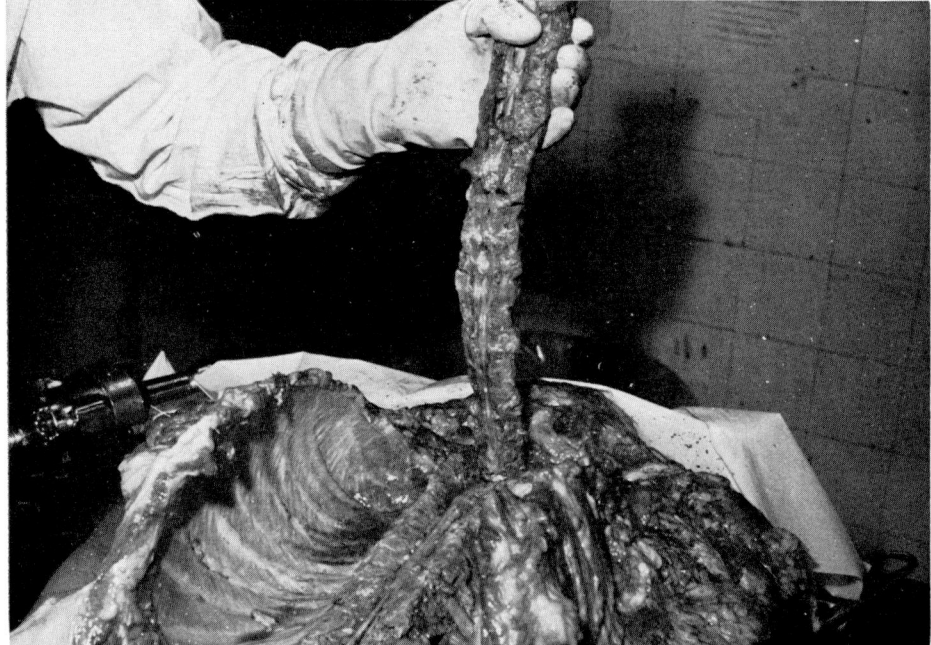

Figure 61. Removal of the column of vertebral bodies.

With the exception of the upper cervical segments, the entire spinal cord within its dural sac and the dorsal root ganglia in their intervertebral foramina are now exposed. If some levels have been cut at too shallow a depth, the excess bone may be taken off with bone forceps. The dural envelope is grasped with a toothed forceps at the L-5 level and, along with the

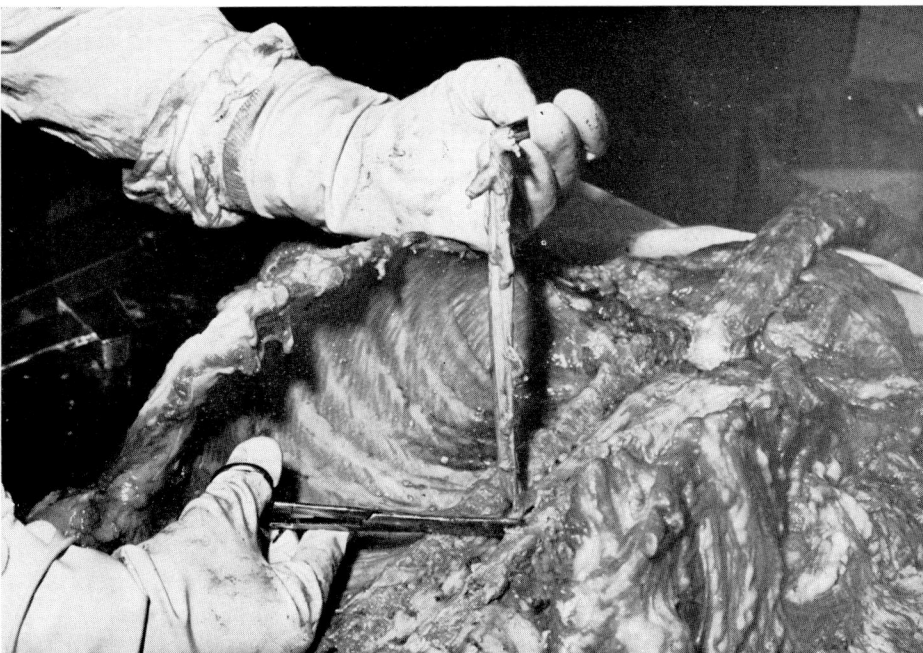

Figure 62. Removal of the spinal cord, alternately transecting roots on the left and right side.

roots of the lower cauda equina, transected. If for some reason the sacral roots and ganglia are also desired for study, the sacrum must be unroofed anteriorly in a manner similar to the rest of the vertebral column.

Holding the lower end of the dura with the forceps and applying slight upward traction, each spinal root is transected distal to the ganglion, if possible. This process is continued from below upward, alternating sides, until the upper level of the vertebral removal is reached.

Now only the short segment of cervical spinal cord within the upper few cervical vertebral segments remains to be removed. This is most readily accomplished in the following manner. With small scissors, the dura at the highest level of the exposed cord is opened transversely and then cut around its entire circumference. When this is done, only the few remaining thin, radicular filaments and dentate ligaments hold the cord in place. A gentle tug downward on the cord will usually free it. Great care must be taken not to squeeze the cord while performing the latter maneuver. If any more than very slight resistance is met in freeing the cord, one should cease tugging immediately. The cervical roots and dentate ligaments are then severed by passing a thin, sharp blade from above, through the foramen magnum, down each side of the cord. When this is accomplished, virtually nothing is holding the cord in place, and it may be pulled free from below, as described earlier.

It is sometimes important to be able to identify specific levels of the spinal cord when it is sectioned following fixation. For this reason it is wise to tag one or two roots which can be used as starting points for counting segments at the time of autopsy when they are most reliably identified.

Ideally, the spinal cord should be fixed in the straight position and not coiled in the bottom of a brain bucket. A catheter tray is most suitable for this purpose. The same formalin solution that is used for brain fixation is used to fix the spinal cord.

NERVE AND MUSCLE

Extensive random sampling of peripheral nerves and skeletal muscle is impractical as part of a routine autopsy procedure. It is customary to sample an easily accessible skeletal muscle, such as the iliopsoas, or nerve, such as the sciatic. When clinical information suggests a disease process involving spinal nerves and skeletal muscles, those which are thought to be affected should be identified and portions removed for histologic study.

A meaningful pathologic evaluation of muscle and nerve requires that as little artifact of manipulation as possible be induced during removal and that sections for microscopy be obtained in planes precisely transverse and precisely longitudinal to the axis of the fibers. Nerve and muscle that has been squeezed or stretched, or is cut at odd angles to the fiber axis, is extremely difficult to evaluate.

In sampling muscle, a longitudinal incision 2 to 3 inches long is made through the skin overlying the belly of the muscle. Two parallel longitudinal incisions, about ¾ of an inch apart and 2 inches long, are made deep into the belly of the muscle. The strip of muscle between these two incisions is then undermined with a third incision. The strip of muscle is now freed except for its ends. A piece of strong thread is passed under the muscle strip near each end and tied tightly. This muscle segment is then severed at each end so that the threads remain attached, and it is lifted out by the threads. It is placed upon a tongue depressor or piece of cardboard cut to a similar shape, and the ends of the thread are tied in such a way that the muscle will be maintained at a constant length during fixation. The muscle is identified by marking the tongue blade in pencil, and it is then placed in formalin solution for fixation. Sections for microscopy will obviously be taken from the central portions of the strip, away from the tied ends.

Peripheral nerves are sampled in an identical manner except, of course, the whole nerve trunk is generally taken, rather than an undermined strip of nerve.

DEFINITIVE GROSS EXAMINATION OF THE BRAIN AND SPINAL CORD

After a period of 10 to 14 days in formalin, the brain is thoroughly fixed. Additional periods of immersion will usually not increase the hardening of brains, especially those softened by autolysis which occurs when the autopsy is delayed after death or, often, if the patient was maintained on ineffective mechanical ventilation for a period of time prior to the certification of death.

The dura over the convexities, which was fixed with the brain, is inspected for external abnormalities. The dura is then removed by folding it back along the midline and cutting the arachnoid granulations, bridging veins along the superior saggital sinus with a scalpel. The dura, including the falx cerebri and tentorium cerebelli, is pulled off. The pineal gland may remain adherent to the tentorium cerebelli and may be pulled away with it.

After inspecting the surfaces of the dura, the superior saggital sinus should be transected at intervals, in search of obstructing lesions.

An orderly inspection of all surfaces of the brain is now conducted. Significant external abnormalities should be photographed before the brain is cut.

If occlusive vascular disease or aneurysm was suspected clinically or is suggested by external abnormalities, the circle of Willis may be removed prior to sectioning the brain. Without undue manipulation of cerebral tissues, the anterior, middle, and posterior cerebral arteries can be transected with scissors 1 to 2 cm beyond their origins. The circle, along with the vertebral and basilar arteries and the proximal segments of the cerebellar arteries, is then easily removed by snipping perforating arteries as they are encountered. The major arteries are then partly transected at frequent intervals with a sharp scalpel, and the cut surfaces are inspected for occlusions. It is wise not to completely transect the arteries until one is actually

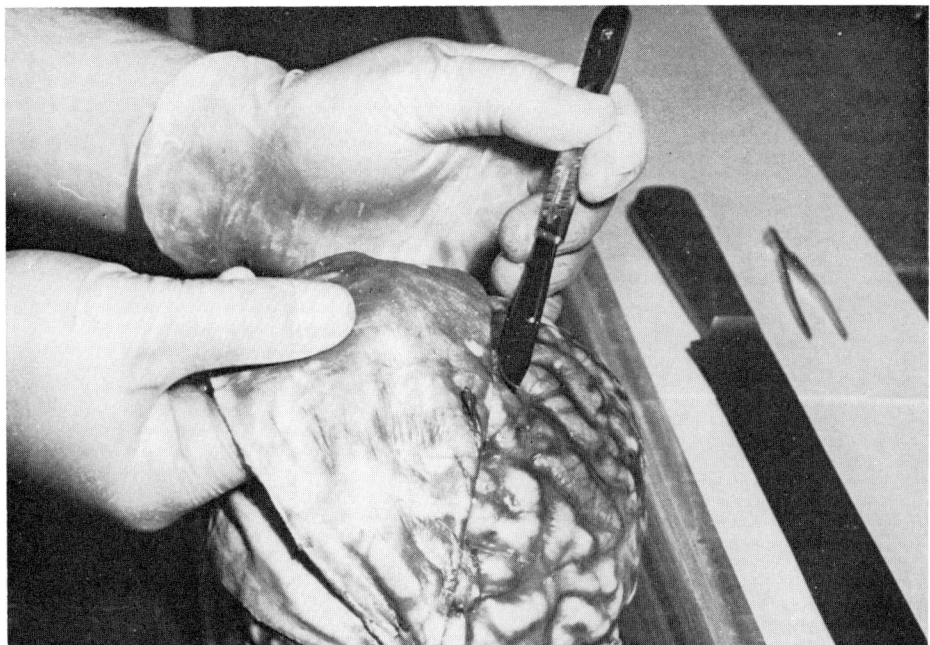

Figure 63. Removal of the dura.

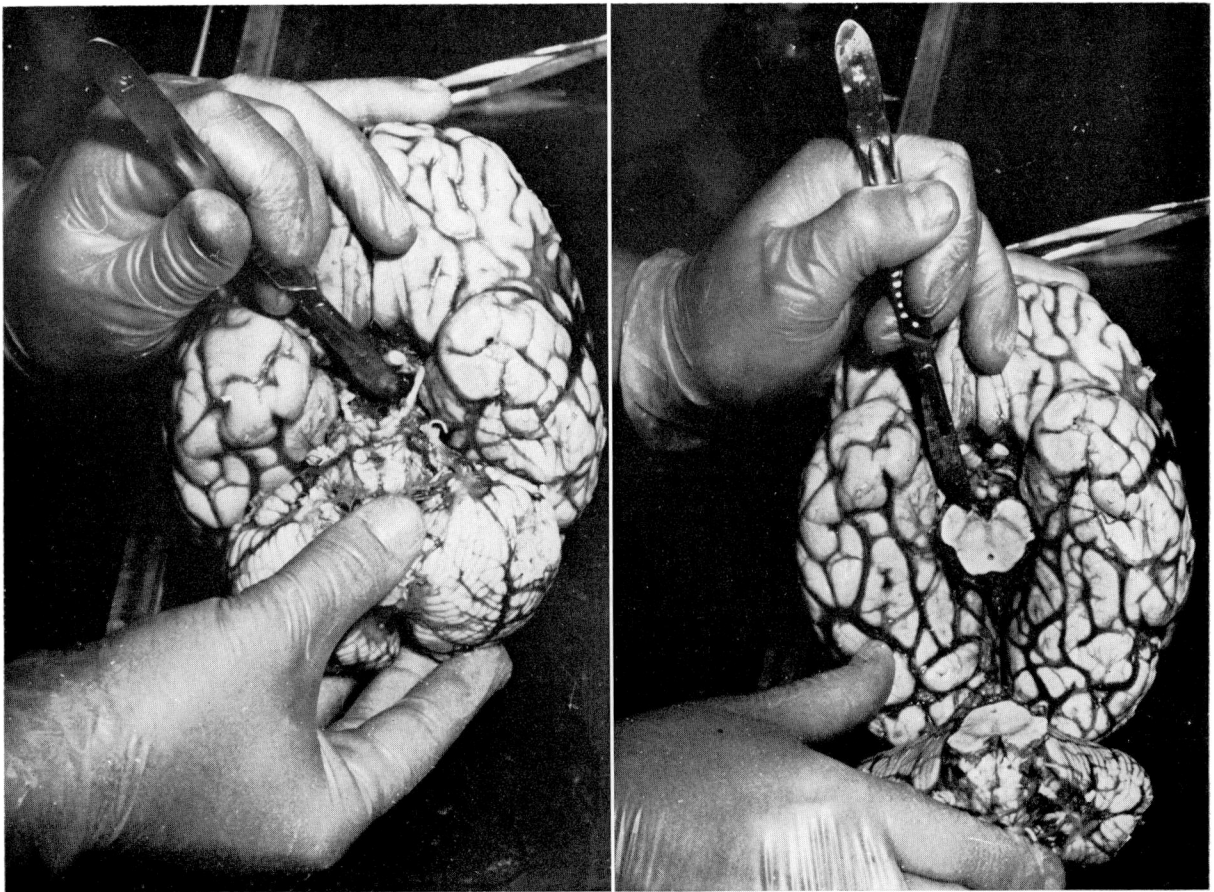

Figures 64 and 65. Removal of the brainstem from the cerebrum.

preparing to submit a clearly identified segment for histologic processing, since important segments may become lost or mixed up.

The cerebral hemispheres are separated from the brain stem by sectioning through the midbrain in the manner illustrated. The scalpel should be directed exactly perpendicular to the long axis of the brain stem and pass through the cerebral peduncles immediately cephaled to the plane of exit of the oculomotor nerves. In order to obtain a flat surface suitable for histologic sectioning, it is extremely important that the transection be made with a single sweep of the scalpel blade. This is accomplished by passing the blade, sharp edge facing medially, directly through one side of the midbrain with a stabbing motion and then, without altering the plane of the blade, bringing it directly across through the opposite side.

The brain stem and cerebellum are set aside, and the cerebrum is prepared for sectioning. Under ordinary circumstances, the custom of sectioning the cerebral hemispheres in the coronal plane at approximately 1 cm intervals is followed. The desired result of this procedure is to obtain bilaterally symmetrical, flat-surfaced, 1 cm thick brain slices. The method whereby this is accomplished is of secondary importance. An exceptionally adept operator may be able to accomplish it "freehand." However, we have found that more consistent and uniform results are obtained with the use of a cutting board, a variety of which are available commercially. The model in use in this laboratory consists, in essence, of a trough with sides that are raised 1 cm. The brain, placed in the trough, is cut by sliding the knife on the raised sides, thus obtaining a 1 cm thick slice. The cutting is usually begun at the frontal pole. The knife used should be very sharp and long enough so that the brain may be cut with one or two long strokes. "Sawing" is to be avoided.

There are several possible approaches to the sectioning of the brain stem and cerebellum. The one which we consider preferable under ordinary circumstances is to section the brain stem and cerebellum together in the plane perpendicular to the long axis. The specimen is held with the left hand cupped under the cerebellum, the ventral surface of the brain stem up, and the thumb steadying the cut surface of the midbrain. The knife blade is

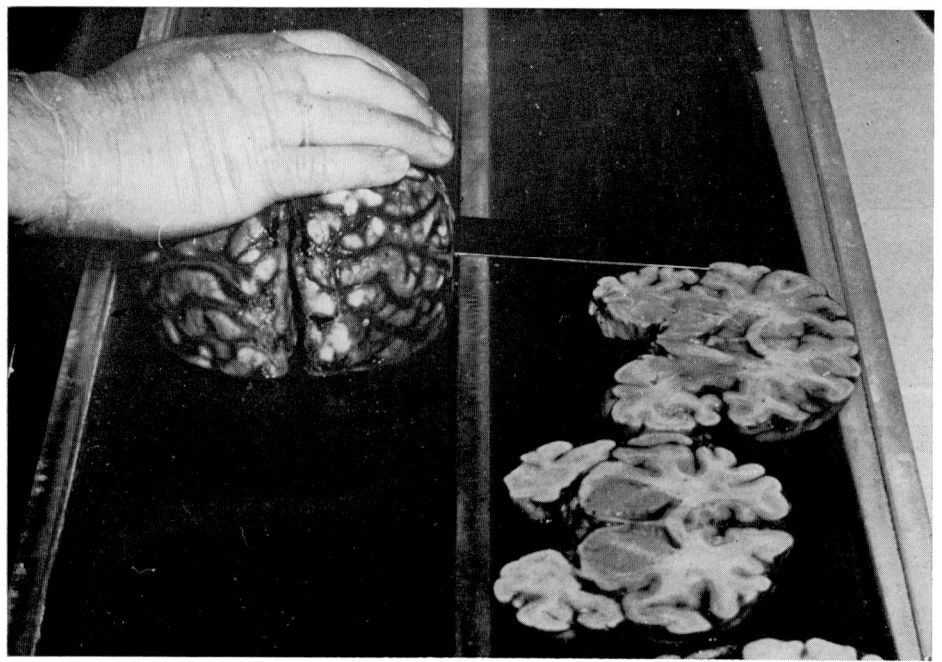

Figure 66. Sectioning the cerebrum into coronal slices, 1 cm thick, on the cutting board.

The Nervous System

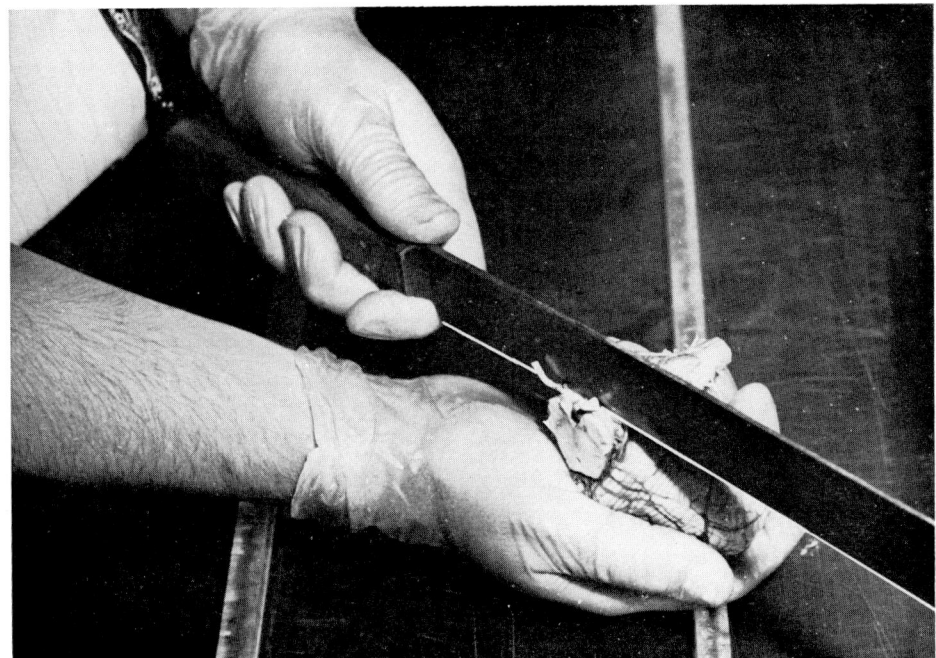

Figure 67

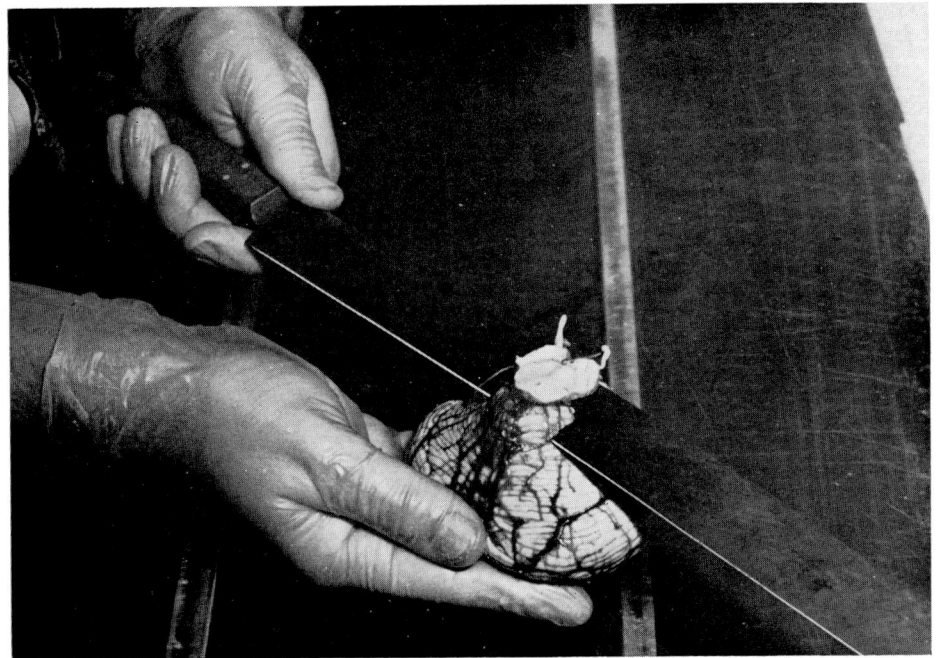

Figure 68

Sectioning the brainstem and cerebellum into coronal slices.

placed exactly perpendicular to the long axis of brain stem, and sections are made at 5 mm intervals. Each cut is begun holding the specimen as described. When the blade has passed approximately halfway through, the grip is changed so that the thumb is moved out of the path of the blade, and the section is completed. The process is repeated at 5 mm intervals down the length of the brain stem and cerebellum in a cephalocaudal direction until the inferior cerebellar peduncle is passed. At this point the small remaining segment of medulla will be free of the cerebellum and the sectioning is completed by placing it on a flat surface and cutting with a scalpel.

It is not possible in microscopic sections to distinguish the left and right sides of the brain stem. Therefore, at some point in the proceedings, before sections are submitted, a microscopically identifiable lateralizing mark should be placed on the brain stem. The method used used in this laboratory is to make an incision no more than 1 mm in depth along the right side of the brain stem.

An alternative method of dealing with the brain stem and cerebellum is to remove the cerebellum from the stem by sectioning the three cerebellar peduncles on each side. The brain stem is then sectioned at 5 mm intervals in the usual plane. The cerebellum is sectioned in the sagittal plane. Certain types of cerebellar disease, particularly those involving degeneration of the vermis, are more clearly demonstrated by this method.

When sectioning is complete, the entire brain is laid out in an orderly fasion and each slide is surveyed for abnormalities. The appearance and location of gross lesions should be recorded verbally and, when possible, photographically.

Although it is a common practice, a system of "routine" sections for microscopic examination is difficult to justify. On the other hand, even in the absence of a history of neurologic dysfunction, almost all disease processes or circumstances which lead to death may cause or be accompanied by microscopic changes in the brain. The lesions which accompany some of the common circumstances associated with fatal illness often occur in characteristic locations such as the "senile changes" that are routinely found in the hippocampus in elderly patients and the hypoxic changes that are frequently found in the hippocampus and other vulnerable areas as a result of preterminal cardiac or respiratory dysfunction. Therefore, sections of one or more of these areas is indicated in almost every brain examined.

Naturally, sections of macroscopically visible lesions should be taken and a record kept of the area from which the tisues was removed. As a general rule, all sections should include some normal-appearing tissue bordering the lesion. Not only does this facilitate microscopic identification of the tissue, but usually the borders of most types of lesions are histographically more interesting and informative.

Sections for microscopy are taken in the following manner. The brain slice from which the section is to be taken is placed in a flat surface. Using a large knife, the entire slice is undercut at a depth of 3 to 4 mm until the area desired for study has been undercut. When the lesion is deep within the brain, better results are usually obtained by undercutting large areas of surface of the brain slice than by attempting to whittle sections from the center of the slice. When the desired area has been undercut, a section of the appropriate size and shape is marked off with scalpel incisions and lifted out.

The examination of the spinal cord is begun with inspection of the external surfaces of the dural envelope. At times, it may be desirable to section the cord within the dura, when, for example, extensive tumor occupies the subarachnoid space. Usually the dura should be opened for inspection of the surface of the spinal cord. Longitudinal incisions are made using scissors along the entire length of the dura in the anterior and posterior midlines. Separating the leaves of the incised dura, the anterior and posterior surfaces of the cord and the intradural spinal nerve roots including the cauda equina, may be inspected and gently palpated. With a sharp scalpel, transverse sections are then made through the spinal cord at 1 cm intervals and the cut surfaces inspected.

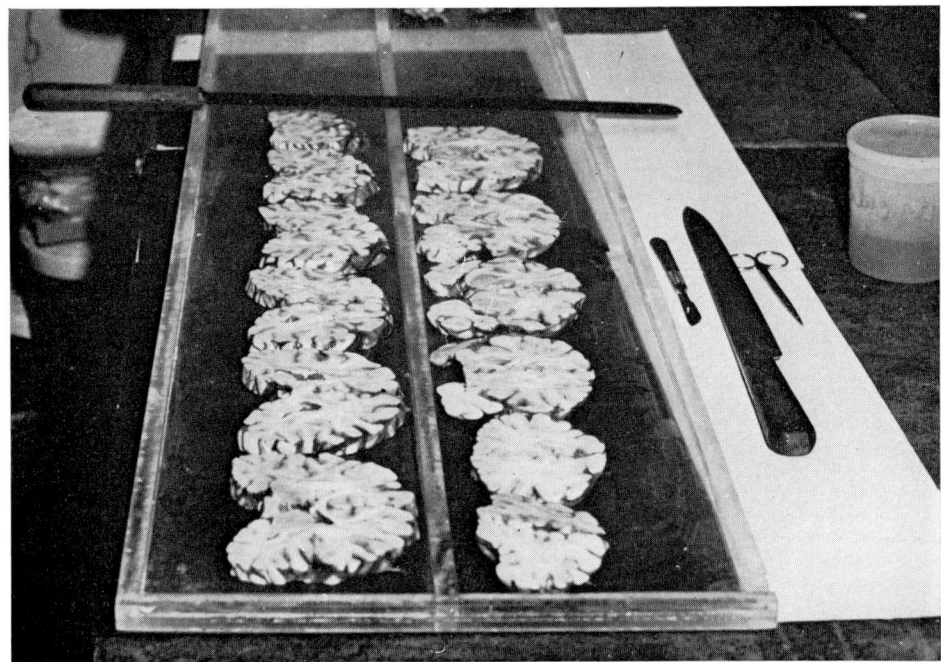

Figure 69

Sections for microscopic examination, 3 to 4 mm thick, are taken from abnormal areas. The precise level from which the section was obtained is determined by counting from the root levels that were identified and tagged at autopsy. As in the case of brain stem sections, a microscopically identifiable lateralizing mark should be etched in spinal cord sections.

Dorsal root ganglia are obtained for sectioning in the following manner. The appropriate intradural root is traced across the subarachnoid space to its point of penetration of the dura. The root is transected in the subarachnoid space and a small window is cut out of the dura around the existing root. The specimen, thus obtained, consists of the subarachnoid portion of the root, a collar of dura, the dorsal root ganglion, and whatever portion of the extradural root was removed at autopsy. Sections for microscopic examination are usually informative when made in the longitudinal axis of this specimen.

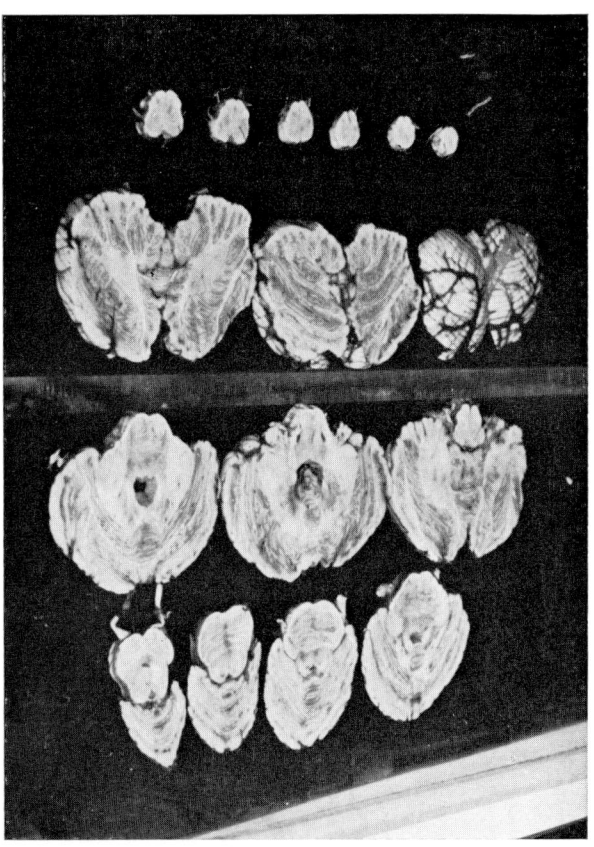

Figure 70

Sections of the cerebrum and brainstem and cerebellum laid out for examination.

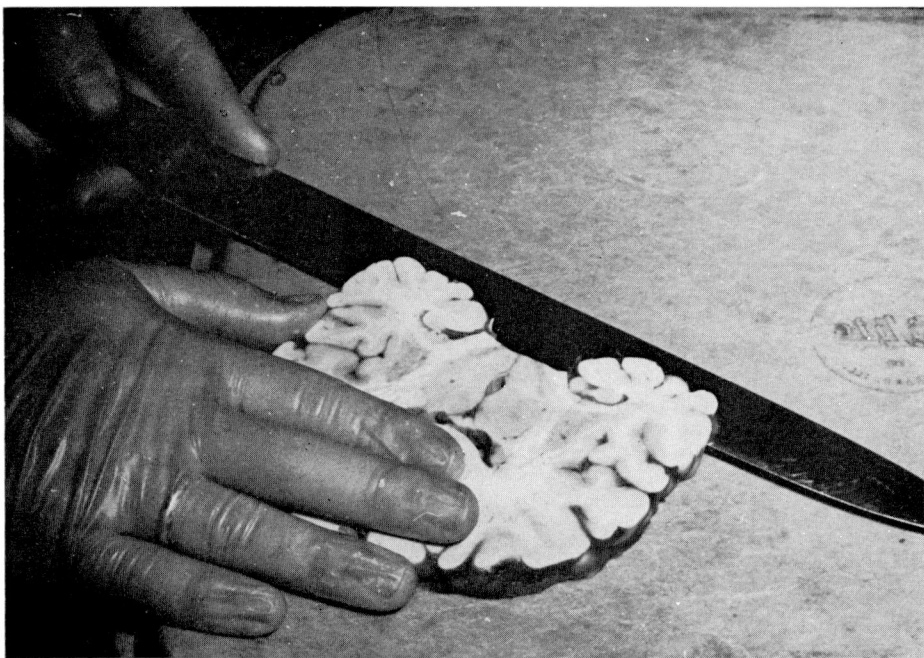

Figure 71. Undercutting the area of a brain slice from which sections will be taken.

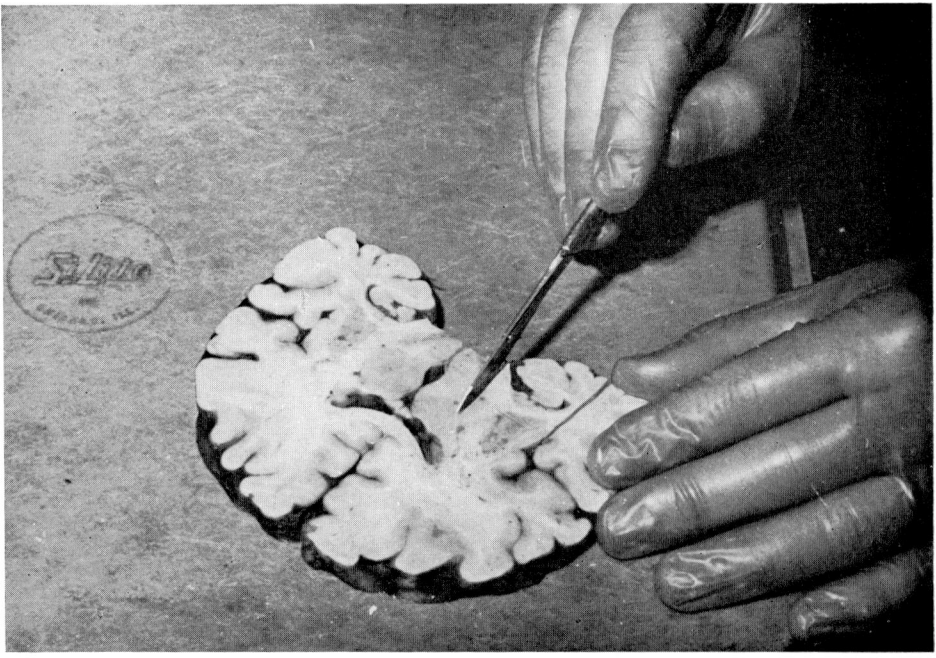

Figure 72. Removing a portion of the undercut area for histologic processing.

Chapter 4

SPECIAL PROCEDURES

DETECTION OF AIR EMBOLI

WHERE air embolism to the heart is suspected, special care must be taken to demonstrate the presence of air in the right ventricle. The opening of the rib cage is now modified so as to maintain the integrity of the internal mammary vessels. The skin flap covering the neck is not reflected so as to prevent introduction of air to the right ventricle which might follow upon accidental section of these vessels if the neck flap were made.

The skin of the chest is dissected free and the rib flap is made lateral to the course of the internal mammary vessels. The rib plate is cut only to the second rib; it is then lifted upward and held by an assistant. The pericardium is opened, and the heart is examined *in situ*. Special attention must be paid to the presence of right ventricular bulging, which is often caused by the presence of massive quantities of air in the heart.

A 30 cc syringe is filled to the halfway mark with water. The syringe must now be tested to see that it is airtight. This is done by testing the connection between the needle base and the syringe nipple. The syringe plunger is now advanced until a stream of water exists and no air bubbles are seen to rise.

The syringe is now introduced into the right ventricle; if air is present it will bubble up in the syringe. With air emboli demonstrated, their source must now be found. If the case in question is a surgical case, the operative area must be inspected to show ligatures which have failed to hold. If the air emboli have risen from rapid decompression following submersion in water, the task is made more difficult. Air embolism occurs under such conditions from decompression often accompanied by mechanical failure of scuba equipment offering increased resistance to the expanding volume of air. Following the law of Boyle, the air expands as pressure decreases. This causes acute pulmonary emphysema, with tearing of the pulmonary parenchyma, hemorrhage, and air entry into the pulmonary vasculature, with resultant air emboli. The cause should under these conditions be sought in a thorough examination of the scuba equipment and in pulmonary sections.

ESOPHAGEAL VARICES

Where it is desirable to demonstrate esophageal varices, a special technique is available. A probe is secured to a string which is approximately 18 inches long. The string is fastened by its other end to the uppermost portion of the esophagus. The probe is now dropped down the lumen of the esophagus and manipulated out through the duodenum. Gentle traction now placed on the probe causes the inversion of the esophagus and stomach, so that the mucosal surface becomes the outer surface. In this manner the esophageal vessels are kept intact and the varices can be visualized. It is advisable to fix the entire block prior to sectioning.

THE THORACIC DUCT

The thoracic duct is located anteriorly to the thoracic vertebra to the left of the azygos vein and to the right of the thoracic aorta. The esophagus lies anteriorly to the thoracic duct. At the level of the third or fourth thoracic vertebra it turns to the left coursing to enter to the left subclavian or innominate vein.

The thoracic duct may be displayed by lifting the right lung up and to the left. In so doing the mediastinal structures are shifted toward the left and the duct is made evident. The right lung, which is effectively serving as a lever here, should not be removed until the thoracic duct dissection is accomplished.

The cisterna chyli, which receives the abdominal lymphatic drainage, is found in the abdomen just below the aorta. It passes with the aorta through the aortic hiatus of the diaphragm to continue into the thoracic duct.

NEONATAL AUTOPSY

This area is one for which entire books have been written. For our purposes, there are only a few points that need be made.

One of the most important observations in the performance of any newborn autopsy is the appearance of the placenta and umbilical cord. How many cotyledons are there, and what are the appearances of the cotyledons of the placenta? Is there any suggestion of infection? Even if there be no gross evidence of placental abnormality, several sections should be made. It is important to inspect the umbilical cord, because several clinical syndromes have now been associated with abnormal vasculature of the cord.

Measurements are made of crown to heel length and crown to rump length. Measurements are also made of head circumference and chest circumference. There are several textbooks in which normal dimensions are given.

It is necessary to examine the head for evidence of trauma, usually manifest by hematomas, for the size of the anterior and posterior fontanelles and the degree of tension of the overlying skin, although this is only reliable if the infant had died within a very short time before autopsy. Careful inspection of the head is made for the presence of Mongoloid facies, abnormalities of the nose and mouth, and of the level and structure of the ears. Does the child have Potter's facies?

The head in neonates is most easily opened with scissors opening along the suture lines rather than the usual method of removing a segment of the calvarium as in adults, with the possible exeption of children with osteoporosis.

The length of the neck is noted as well as the presence or absence of tumors, congenital cysts, or other abnormalities. The chest is first examined for the presence of cutaneous or subcutaneous abnormalities seen with the functional production of so-called "witches' milk." The chest is opened under water, searching for pneumonia in one of two ways. Either the entire body is submerged in a basin of water before opening the chest, or the skin flaps of the chest dissection are reflected and the resultant spaces are filled with water with the chest opened by a scalpel incision below the water level.

The abdomen is inspected for the presence or absence of normal musculature. The genital tract must be carefully examined before evisceration. If there be any evidence of boney abnormalities, roentgenographic examination of the entire body is indicated.

It is very often helpful to remove the chest block intact in the case of neonatal or intrauterine death, thus attempting to maintain not only the relationships between the heart and great vessels, but also between the heart and the lungs. The great vessels are opened carefully within this block, noting origins and disposition of each. The heart is opened by a series of small incisions into each chamber, searching for patency of the interatrial septum, ventricular septal defects, and abnormalities of the associated vessels.

EMBALMED BODIES

Embalmed bodies are extremely difficult to autopsy, not because technical procedures are any different from those used in the non-embalmed, but because interpretation of findings is quite difficult. Whenever possible, such autopsies should be performed by forensic pathologists, even where the case is not of legal importance. We feel that the forensic pathologist is more expert with this type of autopsy as it often constitutes an area of greater experience, due to the fact that exhumed and embalmed bodies are often autopsied for forensic reasons.

Care should be taken in interpretation of findings. Little if anything can be said about skin texture or consistency. Livor mortis is altered by coloring agents which are present in embalming fluids. Rigor mortis cannot be evaluated with reliability. As embalming is performed by the installation of preservative fluids into the body cavities and organs, the points of entry should not be interpreted as lesions. Trochar marks may be found in the organs, and these should be recognized for what they are. Body fluids present in these cavities cannot be evaluated as they are altered quantitatively and qualitatively by admixture of embalming fluids.

The organs themselves show a greyish-red discoloration and are like old rubber, both elastic and brittle. Color differences normally used in the differential diagnosis of diseases are not employable in embalmed organs. Textural differences, although employable in the evaluation of embalmed organs, may be appreciably different from those seen in nonembalmed organs. An example of these differences is seen in the diverse characters which infarcts of the lung have in embalmed and nonembalmed organs. In the nonembalmed lung, an infarct can be described as a firm, well-demarcated, wedge-shaped structure which, on cut section, is shown, dry, granular, and surrounded by a hyperemic halo. In as much, the infarct is most often produced by a thrombus blocking the vessels. In an embalmed body the embalming fluid will be blocked from entry into the infarcted area, consequently the infarct will be soft, depressed, friable, and the hyperemic halo surrounding it will have been diluted by the embalming fluid.

With the exception of those cases in which vascular blockage has occurred, the brain is generally preserved and lesions are easily interpreted.

Where the general pathologist is called upon to perform an autopsy on an embalmed body, his notes should be extensive, and photographs of all organs should be taken so that he may consult with those more expert in the field at a later time if the need should arise.

DECOMPOSED BODIES AND POSTMORTEM CHANGES

As with embalmed bodies, autopsy of decomposed bodies is a field filled with traps for the inexperienced. We will here present a brief review of the sequence of events occurring in the decomposiiton of a body and, where possible, comment on their meaning and interpretation.

Rigor Mortis

Rigor mortis, meaning the rigidity of death, occurs as a result of the interruption of the metabolism of muscle. Provided that an alkaline environment is present in the muscle, as is the case for a short time after death, rigor does not take place. As the environment of the muscle becomes progressively more acid, rigidity begins to occur. At an ambient temperature of 72 degrees Fahrenheit the alkaline environment is maintained for about 2 hours. After approximately 2 hours, muscle glycogen is converted to various acids, and rigidity begins to take place. It occurs first in the facial muscles and progresses in a downward direction to involve the lower extremities at about 12 hours. Rigor persists for a period varying from 12 to 48 hours, and then begins to disappear in the same sequence in which it appeared. The disappearance is due to the reestablishment of an alkaline environment within the muscles subsequent to new chemical changes occurring. In cases in which muscular activity has been great immediately prior to death, rigor will be accelerated in onset. In warm environments rigor is accelerated and its disappearance hastened. Cold thickens the onset of rigor and slows its disappearance.

Livor Mortis

Livor mortis is defined as the bluish-purple discoloration seen in the dependent parts of the body after death. It is due to the settling of blood by gravity after the cessation of circulation. The site of lividity is determined by the position of the body. A body lying face up will develop livor over the back and buttock, whereas a body lying on its side will develop livor on the side on which it is lying. A body lying face down will develop livor over the face, chest, and anterior surfaces of the thighs. When postmortem rupture of blood vessels occurs, small spots of blue hemorrhage occur; this is dependent upon blood volume in relation to capillary size. Lividity begins from 20 minutes to 3 or 4 hours and is usually complete at 2 hours.

The color of the lividity depends upon the proportion of oxygenated hemoglobin to reduced hemoglobin. Carboxyhemoglobin imparts a distinct cherry-red color to the lividity. In bodies exposed to extremities of cold in which peripheral vasoconstriction has occurred prior to death, lividity may be quite pale. Putrefaction changes the color of lividity, as does mummification and, as previously mentioned, embalming. When death is caused by poisons the lividity shows altered colorations.

Putrefaction

Once death has occurred, bacteria normally present in the body, and in the case of infectious diseases, the bacteria responsible for the infection, may proliferate unimpeded. The bacteria gain entrance into vascular structures and pass directly through organs, spreading in this fashion throughout the body of the deceased. Welch bacillus may invade the body shortly after death, the new anaerobic environment favoring their proliferation. Hydrogen sulfide produced in the colon following death reacts with hemoglobin breakdown products to produce the greenish discoloration seen in the bowel and structures in contact with the bowel. This produces a greenish discoloration of the abdominal wall between 1 and 2 days following death. As the blood begins to break down in the postmortem period, it stains and discolors the vessel wall making the subcutaneous vessels very evident. The adipose tissue liquifies and becomes rancid. The brain liquifies; the organs are destroyed. The uterus, prostate, muscle, and bone are relatively resistant, persisting longer than do the parenchymatous organs. When post-mortem gas formation occurs, the body becomes bloated and swollen. The face, abdomen, and genitalia of the male initially show the greatest deformity. Gas formation causes blistering of the skin, and these blisters may rupture causing exfoliation of the skin in irregular sheets. When the skin is exfoliated, irregular areas of fat decomposition are noted as wax-like zones. This is favored by heat and moisture. Conditions favoring decomposition are warmth and humidity. Conditions hindering decomposition are cold and dry environments.

When a body is kept in a cool, dry environment, loss of water is favored. Such environments are provided by sandy soil and well-insulated burial vaults. The skin becomes shrunken and dark in color. The entire body becomes brittle and can fall apart with ease. The skeleton, in any case, is very resistant, and may persist for centuries. This process is called mummification.

All of the previously mentioned events occur to a greater or lesser degree and culminate in the final dissolution of the body. The interval of time required depends upon body size, temperature, humidity, and bacterial flora present.

Estimation of the time of death is difficult from evaluation of the above-described events. Often one is better off using other criteria, such as examination of the scene of death. The scene may show dated unopened mail or yield other informtaion of value in making that determination.

Chapter 5

ACCIDENT PATHOLOGY

THE MEDICOLEGAL AUTOPSY

THE medicolegal autopsy differs from the hospital autopsy both in aim and in significance. It is not performed with the objective of a scientific study of the disease process in mind, although this may be a useful by-product of the autopsy. The medicolegal or forensic autopsy serves the law, and it may well be said that the forensic pathologist holds his C.P.C. in the courtroom.

The purpose of the forensic autopsy is the gathering of evidence for adjudication. The forensic autopsy aims to classify death as natural, accidental, homicidal, or suicidal.

In a case of death due to trauma, in which disease is also found to exist, it is the task of the pathologist to determine whether the disease was the cause of death, whether the accident was the cause of death, or if they both worked together to cause death. It may also be asked if the disease was the principal factor to which the accident contributed, or whether the accident was the principal cause of death, with the disease playing a minor role. A simple example would be a person killed in an automobile collision, found on autopsy to have a transsection fracture of the high cervical cord and a peptic ulcer. One is more apt to die from the transection of the cord than from the ulcer. This is but a simple example.

It is strongly urged that the general pathologist not familiar with these problems defer wherever possible to the trained forensic pathologist. In some areas this may be impossible to do in dealing with accident work. When one considers the number of fatal automobile and household accidents which occur annually and the number of trained forensic pathologists available, it is most probable that these autopsies are performed by general pathologists, often with no forensic training.

The following section should serve as a guide for the general pathologist and does not make pretense of being a text on forensic pathology. We will use the automobile accident as a prototype for the purpose of our discussion.

AUTOMOBILE ACCIDENTS

The records of the pathologist begin at the moment he is notified of the accident and called to visit the scene. The time of notification should be recorded, as well as the name of the party making the notification. This will usually be a police official. The time of arrival at the scene should be noted, as well as the name of the ranking police officer at the scene. Upon arrival at the scene the pathologist takes charge of the body. The following factors are to be evaluated at the scene. Although it might seem superfluous, the pathologist must quickly ascertain if indeed the accident victim is dead. The exact position of the body in relationship to the crashed vehicles should be photographically recorded wherever possible. The relationship of the body to other components of the scene such as trees, road signs, etc. should be noted and photographically recorded. The clothing of the deceased should be described. The presence of livor mortis, rigor mortis, and the body temperature are all to be evaluated at the scene. With the examination of the body complete and the necessary photographs taken, the body may then be ordered removed to the place of autopsy. The attention of the pathologist can now be oriented toward the scene. The crashed automobile should be inspected and areas of damage noted for future correlation with lesions found. Distribution of blood in the crash vehicle and in particular at points of impact between the body and the vehicle should be thoroughly scrutinized. If deemed necessary, blood can be removed from the vehicle for typing.

Upon arrival at the autopsy room the clothing should be inspected. Fragments of glass and blood stains should be inspected and described. In cases in which two or more people are thought to have been in the car at the time of the accident and doubt exists as to who was driving, it is often of use to photograph the soles of the shoes so that imprints which might correspond to the control pedals can be recorded. When these imprints are compared to those of the control pedals the driver can often be identified. Another method would be to fingerprint the steering wheel, which, however, most often yields smudged prints after an accident.

The significance of the above will become apparent from the following example. Two men driving home on a Saturday night were involved in an accident with an oncoming car; both men were thrown free of the car and killed. Autopsy revealed that one man had high alcohol blood levels, and that the other man did not have any detectable alcohol present in his blood. Because of the obvious necessity of fixing responsibility for control of the vehicle on one of the two men, shoe prints which had been taken were employed. These resulted in proving that the driver was the party without alcohol blood levels. The finding was subsequently confirmed by police investigation which revealed that the intoxicated man was driven home from a social gathering at which he was seen by many people to be behaving in an intoxicated fashion, by a friend whose behavior was in no way indicative of intoxication. Clothing, after inspection, should be marked for future identification.

The body is now undressed and the autopsy may begin. Identification photographs and fingerprints should be taken in the case of unknown persons. The external description should be meticulous, each lesion described as to location, dimensions, and particularly color and surface character. The presence of a lesion does not necessarily relate it to an accident. The general pattern of the lesions should be described, so that they may be correlated with the mechanisms of the accident.

The general autopsy should be complete. All organs should be described and all pathology recorded. It is only in this way that a final understanding of the accident can be brought about. Toxicological examination should include blood for alcohol, and where any question however small exists as to the use of other drugs, a general unknown should be performed. Blood may be taken for typing.

We recommend the use of the general medicolegal autopsy protocol shown in this work as a standard form for the recording of data in accident investigation.

Although accidents are one of the major causes of death in the United States, the very nature of the event does not lend itself well to experimental investigation. Each accident is a separate and unique event. The only really efficient means of researching the nature of a given type of accident is to correlate data from as many accidents of the same type as is possible. Hopefully, patterns of injury will thus emerge, and means of preventing them will develop.

"The American Registry of Pathology" located at The Armed Forces Institute of Pathology in Washington, D.C., includes in its mission the collection of all information available in regard to trauma. At this facility which serves as a reference point to which material relative to accident pathology may be sent, studies are made of the forces producing injury and of their effects on tissues. Lesions produced in accidents are studied on a histological, cytological, and histochemical level, as well as ultrastructurally. This institute serves as a consultative service in the study of accident pathology. Submitted material is studied and a report is returned to the submitting pathologist.

HOME ACCIDENTS

Any discussion of accident pathology must emphasize the necessity of obtaining adequate circumstantial information. An example of this is shown in the following case history.

The death of a three-year-old male was reported to the medical examiners' office. The medical investigator on the scene found a young male child lying face down in his bed in a bedroom shared with his older brother, a child five years of age. Livor mortis was present over the face, chest, abdomen, and ventral surfaces of the legs. Rigor mortis was complete. The body was at room temperature. There was no evidence of trauma. The child was clad in pajamas. The parents gave the following history. "The child had been well during the previous evening. He went to bed at the usual bedtime. He awoke and was heard to go into the bathroom during the evening. His parents were awakened a few hours later by noise coming from the bedroom. They found the child awake and somewhat agitated. After calming the child he returned to bed." He was found dead in the morning by his parents.

The medical investigator, patiently pursuing his investigation, inquired into the health of the other child and was able to determine from the parents that their other child was suffering from hyperkinesis and was given amphetamines for the condition by his pediatrician. Inspection of the bathroom revealed an empty prescription bottle. The mother stated that on the night prior to the child's death the prescription bottle had been half-full; approximately ten pills were now missing.

The general autopsy revealed visceral congestion. Toxicology reported high blood levels of amphetamines. The child had apparently thought they were candy.

AQUATIC ACCIDENTS

Resort areas are often the sites of drownings. These areas rarely have a forensic pathologist available. The general pathologist now finds himself with one of the great "hot potatoes" of forensic pathology in hand.

How does one proceed with the investigation? First, a thorough circumstantial investigation is begun. Was the deceased a swimmer or was he unfamiliar with swimming and aquatic sports? What were the circumstances under which he entered the water? What was the aquatic environment at the particular time in which he entered the water? Was he accompanied by a friend? If a friend accompanied the deceased, what did he see? Was the deceased in a postprandial state? Was the deceased known to be suffering from disease?

The body should be carefully examined. If drowning occurred in cold water, liver mortis may be pale due to peripheral vasoconstriction. If the water was sufficiently cold, "cutis anserina" may be present. General autopsy usually shows congestion of viscera. The autopsy should include blood from the left and right ventricular chambers. The blood samples are analyzed for chlorides according to the technique of Getler. For the Getler method to be of value, the samples must be taken within 12 hours after death and show a difference of 25 mg% between heart chambers. In salt water drowning the left heart chlorides are greater than the right. The reverse is true in freshwater drowning. Foreign material such as sand, mud, or stomach contents are often aspirated. Water is often found in the stomach and occasionally in the middle ear. Great emphasis has formerly been placed on the presence of diatoms in the lungs. In recent times it has been shown that these may passively gain entry to the lungs of those already dead upon emersion in water.

Where scuba equipment was in use it should

be thoroughly inspected for the determination of malfunction. A common cause of death in scuba diving is nitrogen narcosis occurring as the swimmer goes to increased depths. Solubility increases with increased depth, the gas following Henry's law. Air embolism occurs as the ascent takes place. The volume of the gas expands following Boyle's law. This volume is reduced via the lungs. Any interference with expiration causes back-up of the air in the lungs with acute pulmonary emphysema and air embolism.

Finally, a thorough general autopsy is necessary to eliminate or include competing causes of death. Where findings are equivocal, the cause of death is best left undetermined.

ELECTRICAL ACCIDENTS

Accidental electrocution is another situation that a general pathologist might find himself confronting. Accidental electrocution might occur from contact with defective household appliances, industrial electrical accidents, unexpected contact with high tension wires, do-it-yourself projects, perverse sexual practices, and by lightning.

The diagnosis in this type of injury, especially when dealing with low voltage current, may be completely circumstantial. In dealing with low voltage currents, it is not rare to have no anatomic findings. In such cases the diagnosis will depend upon the findings of defective electrical equipment with which the deceased was in contact. The exclusion of any other cause of death or competing mechanism of death is essential.

In dealing with high voltage currents, burns at the point of contact are often encountered. These are often irregular in shape and histologically show subepidermal splitting, intraepidermal vesiculation, and spindling of epidermal cells.

If the electrocuting current leaves the body over a wide area, exit burns are often not produced, because resistance at any given point is low. If the exit area is confined and resistance is high, a burn may be produced. Similarly, exit burns may be produced in the clothing.

In death from lightning, arborescent configurations are often present on the skin and may be of value. These are thought to be due to disruption of blood vessels. Intense heat produced by lightning dispersion across the skin may cause the clothing to burst.

Chapter 6

AUTOPSY INFORMATION

PROCEDURES FOLLOWING THE AUTOPSY

AT THE conclusion of an autopsy the prosector should check to see that he has all organ weights recorded. The height and weight of the patient should also be recorded. The organs should then be laid out and the protocol completed. If a dictaphone recording is to be made, it should be made in the autopsy room while all the findings are present. This will minimize omissions. If a short or pictorial form is used, it should be filled out in the autopsy room immediately following the postmortem. The prosector should then assure himself that all sections were taken and place the labelled section bottles in their proper places for subsequent processing.

Before leaving the autopsy room the organs should be placed in buckets containing Jores' solution for keeping for organ review conference. Upon leaving the autopsy area the prosector reviews the chart again and compiles a provisional anatomic diagnosis. This is submitted to the secretary so that a copy can be sent to the interested clinicians.

Most teaching institutions hold a daily organ review of the autopsies performed the previous day. Prior to the organ review conference the prosector should prepare a short clinical summary with which to present his case. Where x-rays are of significance to the case they should also be available for review during the conference. It is the usage at our hospital to submit as "rapid sections" any lesions which are of particular interest at the gross conference. These are reviewed at a bimonthly follow-up conference where the case is then again reviewed in brief. Following the organ review conference all significant findings are photographed for use at departmental and clinico-pathological conferences.

After the appropriate period of fixation, usually 24 to 48 hours in formalin, the organ sections are cut down and submitted to histology for processing. Upon receipt of the sections from histology the prosector should then review his protocol and photographs and begin an inspection of his slides. It is not, in our minds, sufficient for an inexperienced pathologist to make such statements as, "The kidney is unremarkable." It is preferable that he show that he has properly analyzed the slide by commenting on each structure presented. An example of a description of an essentially normal kidney follows: "Four slides are examined, two of right and two of left kidney. The capsule appears thin; the glomeruli shows normal structure; endothelium and mesangium are unremarkable; and the capsules are thin and delicate in appearance. An occasional tubule shows a crystal, but this is infrequent. Proximal and distal convoluted tubules, as well as collecting tubules, are unremarkable. Vessels of all sizes are unremarkable in thickness." In this way, with the prosector required to make a thorough evaluation and record it in detail, he will develop the habit of complete examination of each organ and slide.

With all slides reviewed and described the prosector may now formulate a final anatomic diagnosis. There are essentially two ways in which this may be done. One way is to give the F.A.D. an exclusively anatomic format, listing organ systems separately and giving the diagnosis for each organ system. The second way is to develop in the F.A.D. a sequence of events, for example:

1. Chronic ethanolism (clinical 20 years).
2. Cirrhosis of liver (15 years).
3. Ascites, 5000 cc.
4. Splenomegaly.
5. Esophageal varices.
6. Upper gastrointestinal hemorrhage.
7. Ulcer of duodenum.
8. Coagulopathy.
9. Hepatic coma (clinical).
10. Electrolyte imbalance.
11. Wernicke's encephalopathy.

Either system is usable. We feel, however, that in training programs the second system tends to impress upon the young pathologist the sequence of events leading to the exitus.

The final note has two intentions. Primarily, it is intended to serve as a synthesis of clinical findings and pathological lesions. Its second intention is to give the resident a chance to discuss the case in terms of recent literature in the field and by so doing familiarize himself with all aspects of the disease. It is not intended to document errors or to point to deficiencies in treatment. It is our feeling that whatever a pathologist might think of the therapy or management of a given case, he should not use the final note to express opinions of these aspects of the case.

A well-constructed and properly thought-out final note will give a brief review of the clinical findings, a brief review of the anatomic findings, and a discussion of the relationship between the lesions and the pathophysiology produced by them. Secondly, the final note will present a lucid discussion of the pathology of the disease and how the particular case in question differed from other similar cases. A discussion of the literature bringing the reader up to date on current medical and scientific thinking in the field is the desired culmination of the case study.

The case is ready to be presented to the attending for sign out when the microscopic has been written, the final anatomic diagnosis, and final notes have been written, and all cultures and photographs taken are at hand.

Once the case has been reviewed by the attending it is then submitted to the departmental secretaries for final typing and coding.

PROTOCOLS

Essentially two types of protocols are in use: one is a verbal description of the autopsy; the other is a pictorial protocol. There are two types of pictorial autopsy protocols. One is designed for hospital use, the other for forensic use. We will show the dictated protocol and the pictorial autopsy protocol used in forensic investigation.

The dictated autopsy form presented below is the one in traditional use. We prefer to use this form with junior residents who have not as yet developed their full facility of description and observation of pathological material. In order to properly describe, one must carefully observe. Using this system we do not permit such descriptions as "a thrombus is noted in a pulmonary artery." We prefer that a resident state, "A firm, well-structured, adherent thrombus showing prominent lines of Zahn is noted in a terminal radicle of the pulmonary artery branch leading to the anterior-inferior segment of the right lower lobe." We have noticed with the use of the dictated protocol that the young pathologist's ability to describe improves, his descriptions become clear and concise, and above all, the constant repetition of the criteria by which lesions are diagnosed impresses upon his mind the character of the lesions.

The pictorial protocol used here was developed by *The Panel on Autopsy Protocol* at the International Conference on Accident Pathology in June 1968. The goal is to develop a uniform medicolegal protocol which can be used throughout the United States, so that accumulated information can be stored in a central computer. A similar pictorial form which can be used in hospital pathology is produced by Washington Associates Incorporated. Both pictorial protocols reduce the number of words used to a minimum and allow for speedy recording of data. We feel that they are of great help to the already trained pathologist but are of minimum value in the training of pathologists.

FORMAT FOR AUTOPSY PROTOCOL DICTATION

1. Prosector's name. Autopsy accession number. Patient's name. Chart number. Age. Division (Med., Surg., Neuro., etc.). Ward number. Date of admission. Date of death. Date of autopsy.

2. "The autopsy is performed ____ hours after death. Permission for the autopsy which includes (does not include) examination of the cranial contents is granted by (*Name*), the (*Relation*) of the deceased."

3. *External appearance.* Appearance (development, nutritional state, etc.), apparent age, declared age. Estimated body weight, body length. SKIN: color, turgor, scars, incisions, tumors, eruptions, etc. HAIR: color, distribution. EYES: pupils, irides, sclerae, orbits. EARS and NOSE: note any abnormalities. MOUTH: mucosa, teeth. NECK: trachea, veins, masses, etc. CHEST: symmetry, configuraiton. BREASTS: masses, nipples. ABDOMEN: contour, distension, masses, palpable organs, etc. EXTERNAL GENITALIA: penis, testicles, scrotal masses, vulva. EXTREMITIES: edema, clubbing, joints, etc. BACK: decubital ulcers, kyphoscoliosis, etc. RIGOR MORTIS: moderate, marked, absent. LIVOR MORTIS.

4. "The usual Y-shaped and, if cranial contents are included, intermastoid incisions are made."

5. *Abdominal cavity.* Appearance of the peritoneum, fluid (color, character), adhesions. Location, arrangement of peritoneal and retroperitoneal organs. Omentum and mesenteries. Levels (ribs or interspaces) of domes of the hemidaiphragms. Thickness of the panniculus adiposus.

6. *Chest.* Pneumothorax, fluid, adhesions, pleural surfaces, position of the mediastinum, thymus mediastinal nodes (degree of anthracotic pigmentation, tumor, calcification, etc.), pericardial surfaces and contents.

7. *Heart.* Weight, *in situ* contents of the pulmonary artery, chamber size, epicardium, myocardium, coronary arteries (dominance, degree of atherosclerosis, occlusions, calcification, etc.), valves (leaflets, cusps, commissures, chordae tendineae), valve ring circumferences, thickness of ventricular walls, foramen ovale, ductus arteriosus.

8. *Great vessels.* Aorta and major branches (distribution, position, elasticity, dilatation, atherosclerosis, aneurysms, circumference at the level of the diaphragm, etc.), superior and inferior vena cava, femoral, popliteal, iliac, portal veins, etc.

9. *Lungs.* Weight, lobar divisions, pleura, subpleural lymphatics, bronchi (size and distribution, contents, mucosa, etc.), pulmonary arteries (degree of atherosclerosis, thromboemboli), parenchyma (consolidation, infarction, hemorrhage, tumor, calcification, edema, congestion, aeration, cavity formation, elasticity, emphysema, etc.).

10. *Liver.* Size, shape, weight, color, capsule, blood vessels, intrahepatic bile ducts, consistency, preservation of lobular structure, etc.

11. *Gall bladder and ducts.* Serosa, thickness of wall, mucosa, contents, stones, patency of biliary ductal system, etc.

12. *Spleen.* Weight, size, shape, capsule, consistency, trabeculae, red pulp, malpighian bodies, splenic artery and vein.

13. *Pancreas.* Size, shape, color, consistency, lobular structure, pancreatic duct, etc.

14. *Adrenal glands.* Size, shape, color of cortices and medullae, cortical thicknesses, nodularity, degree of autolysis, etc.

15. *Kidneys.* Weight (separately), capules (adherence to cortical surfaces), appearance of cortical surfaces, cortical thickness and color, medullae, corticomedullary demarcation, papillae, calyces, pelves, ureters. Renal arteries (size, distribution, ostia, degree of atherosclerosis, etc.)

16. *Bladder.* Size, shape, contents, dilatation, hypertrophy, mucosa, cellules, diverticulae, stones, ureterovesicle junction, urethra.

17. *Genital organs.* male—prostate (size, nodularity, induration), seminal vesicles (size, contents), testicles (location, size, shape, hydroceles, color, consistency, tumor, etc.), epididymides, vasa deferentia; *female*—ovaries (size, shape, color, consistency, cysts, tumor, etc.), fallopian tubes (adhesions, thickness, patency, etc.), uterus (size, shape, serosa, myometrium, endometrium), cervix, cagina.

18. *Gastrointestinal tract.* Contents, wall and mucosa of esophagus, stomach, duodenum, small intestine, appendix, large intestine, rectum (tumor, ulcerations, fibrosis, perforations, adhesions, etc.), mesenteric lymph nodes.

19. *Spinal column.* Shape, curvatures, vertebral and intervertebral spaces, bone, bone marrow.

20. *Neck organs.* Thyroid (location, size, shape, color, consistency, nodularity), parathyroid (location, size, color, number identified), pharynx, epiglottis, larynx, vocal cords, salivary glands.

21. *Cranial cavity.* Skull (thickness, shape, etc.), dura and leptomeninges, venous sinuses, weight of unfixed brain, blood vessels at base (atherosclerosis, aneurysms, etc.), middle ears and paranasal sinuses, pituitary.

22. *Spinal cord.* Meninges, size, shape, compression, tumor, etc.

Note:
1. Organ descriptions should be complete and include the appearance of all pathological processes.
2. Diagnostic terms in descriptions are to be avoided.
3. Write the P.A.D. and dictate the protocol immediately after finishing the autopsy.

Clinical summary. The dictated clinical summary should be detailed and complete in the form of a regular ward note (present illness, past medical history, family and social history if relevant, physical examination, laboratory data, xrays, EKG, special studies, hospital course, final clinical diagnoses).

MEDICOLEGAL AUTOPSY REPORT

REGISTRY OF ACCIDENT PATHOLOGY
Armed Forces Institute of Pathology
Washington, D.C. 20305

This form is a computer adapted revision of the Protocol developed and presented by the Panel on "Autopsy Protocol", Dr. Russell S. Fisher, Chairman, at the International Conference on Accident Pathology, Washington, D.C., June 8, 1968.

Both the Conference and subsequent revision and production of this form have been supported from a contract (No. FH-11-6595) awarded by the National Highway Safety Bureau, U.S. Department of Transportation, to Universities Associated for Research and Education in Pathology, Inc.

The Computer Services Division and the Scientific Illustration Division of the Armed Forces Institute of Pathology provided support for the computer adaption and the medical diagrams.

The form has been developed in an attempt to bring into general use in the United States, a standard medicolegal autopsy protocol, the data from which can be stored in a centralized computer facility and used for much needed study and analysis.

Autopsy Information

INTRODUCTION AND INSTRUCTIONS

The MedicoLegal Autopsy Report Form is designed to:

(1) permit a check list recording of medicolegal data in detail
(2) allow the placement of all data into a computer for automatic data processing

This form has 15 pages (1-11 are demographic and medical; 12-15 are contributing factors including environmental). Seventeen pages of anatomical diagrams are provided for optional use.

The form should eliminate loss of data including clerical and coding coverage and yet be medically and legally acceptable. Space is provided for "written in" data and additional sheets may be attached. (The numbers appearing in parenthesis are for data processing only and should be ignored by the pathologist).

A COMPLETE REPORT IS REQUIRED. A CHECK MARK MUST BE MADE FOR EACH ENTRY INCLUDING NOT EXAMINED IF NO STUDY WAS MADE.

The following are examples and notes to be observed:

(A) Please include Zip code with address.
(B) Date/Time should be numerals, based on the 24 hour clock.
Example — January 12, 1969 at 1:15 a.m. would be 01/12/69/0115;
June 9, 1969 at 1:15 p.m. would be 06/09/69/1315.
(C) Check marks (✓) should be appropriately and legibly placed.
Example — An appendix examined and found to be normal would appear as:
APPENDIX: (24)__U_ Present-Not Examined   (25)_✓N_ Normal   (26)__A_ Abnormal   (27)__S_ Surg Absence.

The larynx which reveals edema and other unspecified conditions, would be indicated as: Larynx (24)__U_ Not Exam   (25)__N_ Normal   (26) _✓ E_ Edema   (27)__A_ Surg Absence   (28)_✓O_ Other. Appropriate description of "other" would be made in Remarks, section under NECK ORGANS.

(D) For recording the degree of injury, one of two formats appear, (1) the check-mark type (_0_1_2_3_4_), or the write-in type (_°_).
(E) The use of diagrams is optional to the extent that, only the pertinent ones need to be completed.

Comments and/or suggestions as to the improvement of this form should be directed to:

REGISTRAR — Registry of Accident Pathology
Armed Forces Institute of Pathology
Washington, D.C. 20305

MEDICOLEGAL AUTOPSY REPORT

A RESERVED: (2-9) _____   (Attach additional sheets of 8½ x 11 paper as required.)

CASE NO. (10-19) _____ LAST NAME (20-36) _____ FIRST NAME (37-45) _____ MI (46) _____ AUTOPSY NO. (47-56) _____

SOCIAL SECURITY NO.: (57-65) _____

ADDRESS   ESTIMATED DATE & TIME OF DEATH
Street and No.: _____   ZIP Code   Mo   Day   Yr   Time: (24 Hr Clock)
City and State: _____   (66-70) _____   /   /   /   (71-80)

B   PLACE OF DEATH   DATE & TIME PRONOUNCED DEAD
Location: _____   ZIP Code   Mo   Day   Yr   Time: (24 Hr Clock)
City and State: _____   (10-14) _____   /   /   /   (15-24)

RACE: (25) ___ C Caucasian   ___ N Negro   ___ I Indian   ___ M Mongolian   ___ 0 Other _____   ___ U Unknown
SEX: (26) ___ M Male   ___ F Female   ___ U Unknown   AGE: (27-29) _____ Yrs.   (30-31) _____ Mos.
MARITAL STATUS: (32)   ___ M Married   ___ S Single   ___ W Widowed   ___ D Divorced   ___ U Unknown
OCCUPATION: (Specify) _____
    Occupational Category: (33)   ___ 1 Professional   ___ 2 Skilled   ___ 3 Unskilled   ___ 4 Student
                 ___ 5 Military   ___ 6 Retired   ___ 7 Unemployed   ___ 8 Other: _____   ___ 9 Unknown

                MANNER OF DEATH (From Death Certificate)
(34)   ___ A Accident   ___ H Homicide   ___ S Suicide   ___ N Natural   ___ U Undetermined

           PLACE OF INJURY   DATE & TIME OF INJURY
Location: _____   ZIP Code   MO   Day   Yr   Time: (24 Hr Clock)
City and State: _____   (35-39) _____   /   /   /   (40-49)

METHOD OF OBTAINING REPORT: (50) ___ 1 Autopsy   (51) ___ 2 Inspection   (52) ___ 3 Inquiry

           WHERE PERFORMED   DATE & TIME PERFORMED
Location: _____   ZIP Code   Mo   Day   Yr   Time: (24 Hr Clock)
City and State: _____   (53-57) _____   /   /   /   (58-67)

PROSECTOR'S OR EXAMINER'S Name: _____
    Credentials: (68)   ___ N Not a Physician   ___ 0 Physician (Other Than Pathologist)
                        ___ P Pathologost (Not Boarded)   ___ B Pathologist (Board Certified)
    Type of Board: (69) ___ N None   (70) ___ A Anatomic   (71) ___ C Clinical   (72) ___ F Forensic
WITNESS' Name(s): _____ (73) _____ (74) _____
    Identification: Enter proper code from this list in space provided beside each name.
        ___ 1 Physician (Not Pathologist)   ___ 2 Pathologist (No Board)   ___ 3 Pathologist (Board Certified)
        ___ 4 Policeman   ___ 5 Photographer   ___ 6 Recorder   ___ 7 Other: _____
DISPOSITION OF BODY: (75)   ___ B Buried   ___ C Cremated   ___ 0 Other: _____

C   CAUSE OF DEATH (From Death Certificate)

ICDA Code   Diagnosis
(10-14) ___ . ___ Primary (1): _____
_____

(15-19) ___ . ___ (2): _____

(20-24) ___ . ___ Contributing (1): _____

(25-29) ___ . ___ (2): _____

POLICE JURISDICTION: _____
INVESTIGATORS: _____

PAGE 1

| CASE NO. | AUTOPSY NO. |

EXTERNAL EXAMINATION

RIGIDITY

	Absent	Partially Developed	Fully Developed	
JAWS: (30)	A	P	F	
UPPER EXTREMITIES: (31)	A	P	F	
LOWER EXTREMITIES: (32)	A	P	F	

Remarks: _____

LIVIDITY

	Absent	Fully Developed	Remarks
FRONT: (33)	A	F	
BACK: (34)	A	F	
UPPER: (35)	A	F	
LOWER: (36)	A	F	
LEFT: (37)	A	F	
RIGHT: (38)	A	F	

BODY MARKS: (39) ___ N None (40) ___ S Scars (41) ___ T Tatoos (42) ___ Ø Other: _____

Remarks: _____

PRESERVATION

(43) ___ G Good   (44) ___ A Advanced Decomposition   (45) ___ E Early Decomposition   (46) ___ E Embalmed

Remarks: _____

BODY HABITUS

(47) ___ N Normal   ___ Ø Obese   ___ S Slender   ___ E Emaciated   ___ X Undetermined

Weight of Body: (48-50) _____ lbs or (51-53) _____ kg   Length of Body: (54-55) _____ in or (56-58) _____ cm

Remarks: _____

DIAGRAMS USED

(59) ___ X None		(60) ___ I	Brain — R Lat, Sup, L Lat, Inf	
(61) ___ A Full Length Body — Ant & Post		(62) ___ J	Brain — Coronal Sections (Anterior)	
(63) ___ B Full Length Body — R & L Lat		(64) ___ K	Brain — Coronal Sections (Posterior)	
(65) ___ C Body With Skeleton — Ant & Post		(66) ___ L	Cerebellum, Medulla & Spinal Cord	
(67) ___ D Body With Skeleton — R & L Lat		(68) ___ M	Respiratory Sys, Cardiovascular Sys	
(69) ___ E Head, Neck — Ant, Post R & L Lat		(70) ___ N	Alimentary Sys, Biliary Sys	
(71) ___ F Right & Left Hands — Palmar, Dorsal		(72) ___ Ø	Hemopoietic Sys, Urinary Sys	
(73) ___ G Skull — Ant, Post, R & L Lat		(74) ___ P	Male/Female Reproductive Sys	
(75) ___ H Calvarium (Ext, Int), Base of Skull		(76) ___ Q	Endocrine (Thyroid, Adrenals, Pituitary)	

OTHER PICTORIALS: (77) ___ N None   (78) ___ X X-Rays   (79) ___ P Photos   (80) ___ Ø Other: _____

Remarks: _____

SPECIAL INSTRUCTIONS

Supplement with photographs where possible. Attach additional sheets of 8½ x 11 paper as required.

In each instance during external examination, specify <u>exact location</u> of the injury, abrasion, amputation, burn; and <u>degree of contusion</u>, discoloration, hemorrhage, whether pre-existing or acquired. Also give opinion as to possible cause of injury.

In each instance during skeletal examination, specify exact location and type of fracture or dislocation. X-Rays are to be used where possible. Give opinion as to probable direction and magnitude of force causing injury. Available skeletal diagrams should be used.

CASE NO.	AUTOPSY NO.

INTERNAL EXAMINATION

THE DEGREE OF INJURY SHOULD BE ASSESSED AS: <u>1</u> – MILD (Insignificant); <u>2</u> – MODERATE; <u>3</u> – SEVERE (Potentially Fatal); OR <u>4</u> – EXTREME (Obviously Fatal). ORGANS SHOWING SIGNIFICANT PATHOLOGIC CHANGES SHOULD BE PRESERVED.
(Attach additional sheets of 8½ x 11 paper as required.)

D

SKULL

(10) _____ U Not Examined

If examined, enter codes 1, 2, 3 or 4 as described above on proper line to indicate location and type of injury, or enter 0 under "NONE" if there is no injury.

TYPE OF FRACTURE

LOCATION	None	Linear	Depressed	Other	Description
CALVARIUM:					
Left:	(11) ___	(12) ___	(13) ___	(14) ___	
Right:	(15) ___	(16) ___	(17) ___	(18) ___	
ANTERIOR FOSSA:					
Left:	(19) ___	(20) ___	(21) ___	(22) ___	
Right:	(23) ___	(24) ___	(25) ___	(26) ___	
MIDDLE FOSSA:					
Left:	(27) ___	(28) ___	(29) ___	(30) ___	
Right:	(31) ___	(32) ___	(33) ___	(34) ___	
POSTERIOR FOSSA:					
Left:	(35) ___	(36) ___	(37) ___	(38) ___	
Right:	(39) ___	(40) ___	(41) ___	(42) ___	

OTHER LESIONS: _____

BRAIN

The whole brain should be preserved in 10% N. Formalin after tissue is removed for Toxicology.

APPEARANCE: (43) ____ U Not Examined ____ N Normal ____ A Abnormal   WEIGHT: (44-47) _____ gms

ABNORMALITIES: Use a check (√) to indicate location and type

	Contusion	Laceration	Pre-existing Lesion	Remarks
CEREBRUM:				
Left:	(48) ___ C	(49) ___ L	(50) ___ P	
Right:	(51) ___ C	(52) ___ L	(53) ___ P	
CEREBELLUM:				
Left:	(54) ___ C	(55) ___ L	(56) ___ P	
Right:	(57) ___ C	(58) ___ L	(59) ___ P	
MID BRAIN:				
Left:	(60) ___ C	(61) ___ L	(62) ___ P	
Right:	(63) ___ C	(64) ___ L	(65) ___ P	

Remarks: _____

SWELLING:	(66) ___	0	1	2	3	4
ANEURYSM:	(67) ___	0	1	2	3	4
ATHEROSCLEROSIS:	(68) ___	0	1	2	3	4
OTHER ABNORMALITY:	(69) ___	0 Absent		1 present		

E

HEMORRHAGE: (Record volume in cc)

	Left	Right	
Extra Dural:	(10-12) ___	(13-15) ___	
Sub Dural:	(16-18) ___	(19-21) ___	
Sub Arachnoid:	(22-24) ___	(25-27) ___	
Intracerebral:	(28-30) ___	(31-33) ___	
Intraventricular:	(34-36) ___	(37-39) ___	

Remarks _____

CASE NO.	AUTOPSY NO.

INTERNAL (continued)

PITUITARY

(40) ___U___ Not Examined   (41) ___N___ Normal   (42) ___T___ Trauma   (43) ___∅___ Other Pathology:

Remarks: _____

SPINAL CORD

(44) ___U___ Not Examined   (45) ___N___ Normal   (46) _____ Pre-existing Lesion   (47) ___L___ Lacerated

(48) ___C___ Contused   (49) ___T___ Transected   Remarks: _____

MIDDLE AND INNER EAR

LEFT: (50) ___U___ Not Examined   (51) ___N___ Normal   (52) ___P___ Pre-existing Lesion   (53) ___H___ Hemorrhage

RIGHT: (54) ___U___ Not Examined   (55) ___N___ Normal   (56) ___P___ Pre-existing Lesion   (57) ___H___ Hemorrhage

Remarks _____

EYES

	Not Examined	Normal	Trauma	Cataract	Opacity (O)	Other
LEFT:	(58) ___U___	(59) ___N___	(60) ___T___	(61) ___C___	(62) _____	(63) ___∅___
RIGHT:	(64) ___U___	(65) ___N___	(66) ___T___	(67) ___C___	(68) _____	(69) ___∅___

Remarks: _____

ORAL CAVITY

F

TONGUE: (10) ___U___ Not Examined   (11) ___N___ Normal   (12) ___L___ Lacerated   (13) ___∅___ Other:

FRACTURES: (14) ___U___ Not Examined   ___N___ None Present

　Maxilla: (15) ___L___ Left   (16) ___R___ Right   Mandible: (17) ___L___ Left   (18) ___R___ Right

　Dental: (19) ___U___ Upper   (20) ___L___ Lower   Number of Teeth Fractured: _____

PLATES: (21) ___U___ Upper   (22) ___L___ Lower   (23) ___N___ None

Remarks: _____

NECK ORGANS

LARYNX: (24) ___U___ Not Exam   (25) ___N___ Normal   (26) ___E___ Edema   (27) ___A___ Surg Absence   (28) ___∅___ Other

　Hemorrhage: (Record Degree) (29) 1 2 3 4

FRACTURES: (30) ___U___ Not Exam   (31) ___N___ None   (32) ___C___ Cricoid   (33) ___T___ Thyroid   (34) ___H___ Hyoid

THYMUS: (35) ___U___ Not Exam   (36) ___N___ Not Identified   (37) ___P___ Prev Path   (38) ___T___ Trauma

　Weight: _____ gms

THYROID: (39) ___U___ Not Exam   (40) ___N___ Normal   (41) ___P___ Pre-existing Lesion   (42) ___T___ Trauma

　Weight: _____ gms

PARATHYROIDS: (43) ___U___ Not Exam   (44) ___N___ Normal   (45) ___P___ Pre-existing Lesion   (46) ___T___ Trauma

Remarks _____

PLEURAL SPACE

(47) ___U___ Not Examined   ___N___ Normal   ___A___ Abnormal

ABNORMALITIES: Adhesions   Pneumothorax   Hemothorax   Perforated Pleura   Other

　Left: (48) ___1___   (49) ___2___   (50) ___3___ cc   (51) ___4___   (52) ___5___

　Right: (53) ___1___   (54) ___2___   (55) ___3___ cc   (56) ___4___   (57) ___5___

Remarks: _____

| CASE NO. | | AUTOPSY NO. |

INTERNAL (continued)

CHEST WALL

(58) _____ U Not Examined _____ N Normal _____ A Abnormal
SOFT TISSUE INJURY: (59) _____ C Contusion (60) _____ Ø Other: _____
  Size of Wound: Length (61-62) _____ in   Width (63-64) _____ In
FRACTURES: (65) _____ N None   (66) _____ L Left Rib Fx   (67) _____ R Right Rib Fx
  (68) _____ S Sternal   (69) _____ W Unstable Chest Wall
Remarks: _____

TRACHEA

(70) _____ U Not Exam   (71) _____ N Normal   (72) _____ T Trauma   (73) _____ P Tracheostomy   (74) _____ B Blood
(75) _____ M Mucus   (76) _____ V Vomitus/Food   (77) _____ Ø Foreign Object: _____
Evidence of Smoke Inhalation?   (78) _____ Y Yes   _____ N No
Remarks: _____

LUNGS

G

(10) _____ U Not Examined _____ N Normal _____ A Abnormal
WEIGHT: Left (11-14) _____ gms   Right (15-18) _____ gms
ABNORMALITIES: For each condition, check "L" for Left and "R" for Right as appropriate.

Aspirated Blood:	(19) L	(20) R	Laceration:	(21) L	(22) R
Aspirated Vomitus:	(23) L	(24) R	Perforation:	(25) L	(26) R
Aspiration Pneumonia:	(27) L	(28) R	Hemorrhage/Contusion:	(29) L	(30) R
Broncho Pneumonia:	(31) L	(32) R	Atelectasis:	(33) L	(34) R
Lobar Pneumonia:	(35) L	(36) R	Emphysema:	(37) L	(38) R
Edema:	(39) L	(40) R	Thromboembolism:	(41) L	(42) R
Other:	(43) L	(44) R			

Remarks _____

DIAPHRAGM

(45) _____ U Not Examined   (46) _____ N Normal   (47) _____ L Laceration   (48) _____ Ø Other: _____
Remarks: _____

GREAT VESSELS

AORTA: (49) _____ U Not Examined _____ N Normal _____ A Abnormal
  Aneurysm (Thoracic) (50) _1_ _2_ _3_ _4_   Aneurysm (Abdominal) (51) _1_ _2_ _3_ _4_
  Atherosclerosis (52) _1_ _2_ _3_ _4_   Trauma (53) _1_ _2_ _3_ _4_
Remarks: _____
VENA CAVA: (54) _____ U Not Examined   (55) _____ N Normal   Trauma (56) _1_ _2_ _3_ _4_
Remarks: _____
OTHER MAJOR ARTERIES: (57) _____ U Not Examined   (58) _____ N Normal   Trauma (59) _1_ _2_ _3_ _4_
OTHER MAJOR VEINS: (60) _____ U Not Examined   (61) _____ N Normal   Trauma (62) _1_ _2_ _3_ _4_
Remarks: _____

HEART

(63) _____ U Not Exam   (64) _____ N Normal   (65) _____ E Air Embolism   (66) _____ T Trauma   (67) _____ P Pre-exist Lesion
(68) _____ V Valvular Disease   WEIGHT: (69-72) _____ gms   Remarks: _____

| CASE NO. | AUTOPSY NO. |

INTERNAL (continued)

PERICARDIUM

(10) ____ U Not Examined (11) ____ N Normal (12) ____ P Pre-existing Lesion (13) ____ R Rupture
(14) ____ ∅ Other: _____ Hemopericardium: (15-18) ____ cc
Remarks: _____

CORONARY VESSELS

(19) ____ U Not Examined   ____ N Normal   ____ A Abnormal

Assess Maximal Degree of Occlusion as: "1" — Minimum (less than 20%), "2" — Mild (from 20 to 50%), "3" — Moderate (from 50 to 80%) and "4" — Severe (from 80 to 100%).

CHART LOCATION AND DEGREE OF NARROWING

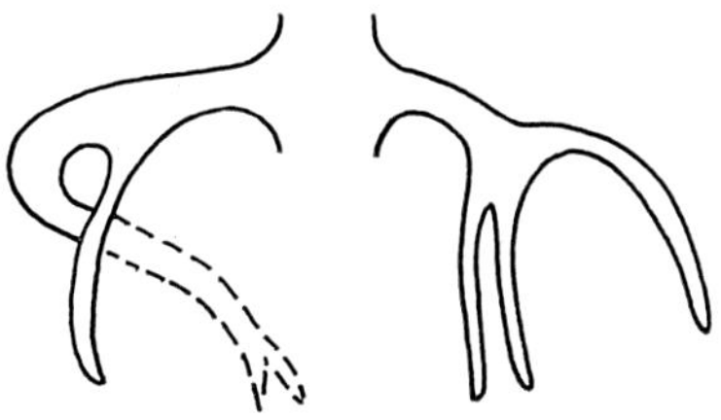

RIGHT: (20) __ 0 __ 1 __ 2 __ 3 __ 4

LEFT MAIN: (21) __ 0 __ 1 __ 2 __ 3 __ 4

LEFT DESCENDING: (22) __ 0 __ 1 __ 2 __ 3 __ 4

LEFT CIRCUMFLEX: (23) __ 0 __ 1 __ 2 __ 3 __ 4

Remarks: _____

MYOCARDIUM

(24) ____ U Not Examined (25) ____ N Normal (26) ____ T Trauma (27) ____ I Infarct (28) ____ ∅ Other

TRAUMA:
    (29) ____ C Contusion   (30) ____ P Epicardial Laceration   (31) ____ N Endocardial Laceration
    (32) ____ R Rupture

MECHANISM OF TRAUMA: (33) ____ G Gunshot Wound   (34) ____ R Rib Perforation
    (35) ____ C Compression   (36) ____ F Foreign Body Perforation

Remarks: (Include description of Mechanism) _____

INFARCT: Specify Location: _____
Classify as "Acute" (Less than 24 Hrs.), "Recent" (1 day to 1½ wk), "Healing" (over 2 wks.)

(37) ____ A Acute: (38) ____ 1 Focal   __ 2 Moderate to Large   __ 3 Massive
(39) ____ R Recent: (40) ____ 1 Focal   __ 2 Moderate to Large   __ 3 Massive
(41) ____ H Healing: (42) ____ 1 Focal   __ 2 Moderate to Large   __ 3 Massive
(43) ____ S Scarring: (44) ____ 1 Focal   __ 2 Moderate to Large   __ 3 Massive

Remarks: _____

OTHER HEART DISEASE: (45) ____ U Not Examined   ____ P Present   ____ A Absent
Description: _____

PERITONEUM

(46) ____ U Not Examined   (47) ____ N Normal
(48) ____ P Pre-existing Lesions   (49) ____ ∅ Other (include contusion of wall)
    Hemoperitoneum: (50-53) ____ cc   Acites: (54-57) ____ cc

Remarks: _____

CASE NO.	AUTOPSY NO.

INTERNAL (continued)

ESOPHAGUS

(58) _____ U Not Examined   (59) _____ N Normal   (60) _____ T Trauma or Laceration   (61) _____ Ø Other Lesions

Remarks: _____

STOMACH

(62) _____ U Not Examined   (63) _____ N Normal   (64) _____ T Trauma or Rupture   (65) _____ P Perforation

(66) _____ Ø Other Lesions: _____   VOLUME OF CONTENTS: (67-70) _____ cc

DESCRIPTION OF CONTENTS: (71) _____ B Bloody   (72) _____ C Coffee Ground   (73) _____ S Bile Stained

   (74) _____ M Mucous   (75) _____ S Serous   (76) _____ M Medication   (77) _____ Ø Other

Remarks: (Specify other, if checked) _____

INTESTINES

SMALL: (including Mesentery) (10) _____ U Not Examined   (11) _____ N Normal   (12) _____ C Contusion

   (13) _____ L Laceration   (14) _____ P Perforation   (15) _____ Ø Other   (16) _____ P Pre-existing Lesion

Remarks: _____

LARGE: (17) _____ U Not examined   (18) _____ N Normal   (19) _____ C Contusion   (20) _____ L Laceration

   (21) _____ P Perforation   (22) _____ Ø Other   (23) _____ P Pre-existing Lesion

Remarks: _____

APPENDIX: (24) _____ U Present-Not Exam   (25) _____ N Normal   (26) _____ A Abnormal   (27) _____ S Surg Absence

Remarks: _____

LIVER

(28) _____ U Not Examined   (29) _____ N Normal   (30) _____ T Trauma   (31) _____ P Pre-existing Lesion

TRAUMA: (Classify as 1st, 2nd, 3rd or 4th degree.)

   Contusion (32) _____°   Laceration (33) _____°   Perforation (34) _____°   Pulpefaction (35) _____°

PRE-EXISTING LESIONS: (36) _____ F Fatty Infiltration   (37) _____ Ø Other   WEIGHT: (38-41) _____ gms

Remarks: _____

SPLEEN

(42) _____ U Present-Not Examined   _____ N Normal   _____ A Abnormal   _____ S Surgical Absence

TRAUMA: Laceration (43) _____°   Perforation (44) _____°   WEIGHT: (45-48) _____ gms

Remarks: _____

GALL BLADDER

(49) _____ U Present-Not Examined   _____ N Normal   _____ A Abnormal   _____ S Surgical Absence

Remarks: _____

PANCREAS

(50) _____ U Not Exam   (51) _____ N Normal   Contusion (52) _____°   Laceration (53) _____°   (54) _____ Ø Other

WEIGHT: (55-58) _____ gms   Remarks: _____

CASE NO.	AUTOPSY NO.

INTERNAL (continued)

ADRENALS

LEFT: (59) ____ U Not Exam   (60) ____ N Normal   (61) ____ H Hemorrhage   (62) ____ L Laceration   (63) ____ Ø Other
RIGHT: (64) ____ U Not Exam   (65) ____ N Normal   (66) ____ H Hemorrhage   (67) ____ L Laceration   (68) ____ Ø Other
WEIGHT: Left (69-70) ____ gms   Right (71-72) ____ gms
Remakrs: _____

GENITO–URINARY SYSTEM

KIDNEY

LEFT: (10) ____ U Present-Not Exam   ____ N Normal   ____ S Surgical Absence   ____ T Trauma
          TRAUMATIC LESIONS: Contusion (11) ____ o   Laceration (12) ____ o   Perforation (13) ____ o
          (14) ____ Ø OTHER LESIONS: _____   WEIGHT: (15-17) ____ gms
RIGHT: (18) ____ U Present-Not Exam   ____ N Normal   ____ S Surgical Absence   ____ T Trauma
          TRAUMATIC LESIONS: Contusion (19) ____ o   Laceration (20) ____ o   Perforation (21) ____ o
          (22) ____ Ø OTHER LESIONS: _____   WEIGHT: (23-25) ____ gms
Remarks: _____

URINARY BLADDER

(26) ____ U Not Examined   (27) ____ N Normal   (28) ____ P Pre-existing Lesions
(29) ____ T Trauma and/or Perforation   (30) ____ Ø Other Lesions   CONTENTS: (31-34) ____ cc
Remarks: _____

(If Subject Is Female, Skip To Next Page.)

MALE ORGANS

PROSTATE

(35) ____ U Not Examined   ____ N Normal   ____ A Abnormal
Remarks: _____

PENIS

(36) ____ U Not Examined   (37) ____ N Normal   (38) ____ A Abnormal   (39) ____ C Circumcision
Remarks: _____

TESTIS

LEFT: (40) ____ U Present-Not Exam   (41) ____ N Normal   (42) ____ S Surg Absence   (43) ____ T Trauma   (44) ____ Ø Other
RIGHT: (45) ____ U Present-Not Exam   (46) ____ N Normal   (47) ____ S Surg Absence   (48) ____ T Trauma   (49) ____ Ø Other
Remarks: _____

| CASE NO. | AUTOPSY NO. |

INTERNAL (continued)

(If Subject Is Male, Skip To Next Page.)

FEMALE ORGANS

UTERUS

(35) _____ U Present-Not Examined (36) _____ N Normal (37) _____ S Surgical Absence (38) _____ P Pregnant

(39) _____ P Post Partum (40) _____ T Trauma: _____ (41) _____ Ø Other Lesions: _____

Remarks: _____

CERVIX

(42) _____ U Present-Not Examined (43) _____ N Normal (44) _____ S Surgical Absence (45) _____ P Pregnant

(46) _____ P Post Partum (47) _____ T Trauma: _____ (48) _____ Ø Other Lesions: _____

Remarks: _____

OVARY

LEFT: (49) _____ U Present-Not Exam (50) _____ N Normal (51) _____ S Surg Absence (52) _____ T Trauma (53) _____ Ø Other

RIGHT: (54) _____ U Present-Not Exam (55) _____ N Normal (56) _____ S Surg Absence (57) _____ T Trauma (58) _____ Ø Other

Remarks: _____

FALLOPIAN TUBE

LEFT: (59) _____ U Present-Not Exam (60) _____ N Normal (61) _____ S Surg Absence (62) _____ T Trauma (63) _____ Ø Other

RIGHT: (64) _____ U Present-Not Exam (65) _____ N Normal (66) _____ S Surg Absence (67) _____ T Trauma (68) _____ Ø Other

Remarks: _____

VAGINA

(69) _____ U Not Examined (70) _____ N Normal (71) _____ A Abnormal (72) _____ L Laceration

Specimen taken? (73) _____ Y Yes _____ N No

Remarks: (Include type of specimen and results) _____

Autopsy Information

	CASE NO.									AUTOPSY NO.	

INTERNAL (continued)

SKELETAL

FRACTURES: (Check all applicable columns — include disc separations.)

TRAUMA: _____

	Location	Not Exam	/	Normal	/	Minor	/	Severe	/	Single	/	Multiple	/	Simple	/	Compound	/	Comminuted
K	Cervical Spine:	(10)___U		(11)___N		(12)__1		(13)__3		(14)__S		(15)__M		(16)__1		(17)__2		(18)__3
	Dorsal Spine:	(19)___U		(20)___N		(21)__1		(22)__3		(23)__S		(24)__M		(25)__1		(26)__2		(27)__3
	Lumbar Spine:	(28)___U		(29)___N		(30)__1		(31)__3		(32)__S		(33)__M		(34)__1		(35)__2		(36)__3
	Pelvis:	(37)___U		(38)___N		(39)__1		(40)__3		(41)__S		(42)__M		(43)__1		(44)__2		(45)__3
	Upper Extremity:																	
	Left:	(46)___U		(47)___N		(48)__1		(49)__3		(50)__S		(51)__M		(52)__1		(53)__2		(54)__3
	Right:	(55)___U		(56)___N		(57)__1		(58)__3		(59)__S		(60)__M		(61)__1		(62)__2		(63)__3
L	Lower Extremity:																	
	Left:	(10)___U		(11)___N		(12)__1		(13)__3		(14)__S		(15)__M		(16)__1		(17)__2		(18)__3
	Right:	(19)___U		(20)___N		(21)__1		(22)__3		(23)__S		(24)__M		(25)__1		(26)__2		(27)__3

PRE-EXISTING LESIONS: Osteoporosis   (28)____ Y Yes   ____ N No

     Other Disease (include tumors)   (29)____ Y Yes   ____ N No

Remarks: _____

_____

_____

HEMOPOIETIC SYSTEM

LYMPH NODES: (30)____   U Not Examined   ____ N Normal   ____ A Abnormal

BONE MARROW: (31)____   U Not Examined   ____ N Normal   ____ A Abnormal

Remarks: _____

_____

BIOCHEMICAL AND TOXICOLOGY

ETHANOL: (32)____ P Performed   ____ N Not Performed   Method: _____

Urine Level: (33-36)____.____ mgm%   (37-39)____.____ %   Blood Level: (40-43)____.____ mgm%   (44-46)____.____ %

Other: (47-50)_____ Specify: _____

Remarks: _____

_____

CARBON MONOXIDE: (51)____ P Performed   ____ N Not Performed   % Saturation: (52-55)_____

Remarks: _____

ANALYSES FOR DRUGS OR MEDICATIONS: (56)____ P Performed   ____ N Not Performed

     FINDINGS: (57)____ B Barbiturates   (58)____ A Amphetamines   (59)____ Ø Opiates   (60)____ T Tranquilizers

     (61)____ A Antihistamines   (62)____ Ø Other: _____

Remarks: (Include type and level) _____

CASE NO.	AUTOPSY NO.

INTERNAL (continued)

BIOMEDICAL AND TOXICOLOGY (continued)

OTHER TOXICOLOGY TESTS:　　(63) _____ P Performed　　　　_____ N Not Performed

　　Results Positive?　　　　(64) _____ Y Yes　　　　　　　_____ N No

Remarks: Specify Findings) _____

_____

_____

_____

BLOOD GROUP: (65) ___ 1 (0+) ___ 2 (0-) ___ 3 (A+) ___ 4 (A-) ___ 5 (B+) ___ 6 (B-) ___ 7 (AB+) ___ 8 (AB-)

Remarks and/or Special Blood Studies: _____

_____

_____

_____

SPECIAL STUDIES

CLOTHING: (66) ___ U Not Examined　　(67) ___ E Examined　　Preserved? (68) ___ Y Yes　(69) ___ N No

Remarks: (Specify Findings and How Clothing Disposed) _____

_____

_____

_____

PHOTOGRAPHS (Available to Pathologist):　(70) ___ 0 None　　(71) ___ 1 Scenes

　　(72) ___ 2 Vehicle　　(73) ___ 3 Victim (external)　　(74) ___ 4 Organ Photographs

Remarks: _____

_____

HISTOLOGICAL FINDINGS

List supplemental Positive Findings. (Use additional sheets of paper if necessary.)

FAT EMBOLISM: (75) ___ U Not Examined　　Degree: (76) _____ °　Organ _____

　　(77) ___ ∅ Other: _____

Remarks: _____

_____

_____

(Space For Additional or Continued Remarks)

_____
_____
_____
_____
_____
_____
_____
_____
_____
_____
_____
_____
_____
_____
_____

| CASE NO. | AUTOPSY NO. |

FACTORS CONTRIBUTING TO ACCIDENT

HUMAN FACTORS

M

PHYSICAL: (Pre-existing Disease)　(10) ___Y__ Yes　　___ No　　__X__ Unknown
　Type:　(11) __1__ Cerebral　(12) __2__ Cardiovascular　(13) __3__ Other (Specify) _____
Remarks: _____

VISION: (14) __N__ Normal　　__A__ Abnormal　　__X__ Unknown
　Spectacles: (15) __W__ Worn　(16) __N__ Not Worn　Contacts: (17) __W__ Worn　(18) __N__ Not Worn
Remarks: _____

HEARING: (19) __N__ Normal　　__A__ Abnormal　　__X__ Unknown
　Hearing Aid: (20) __1__ Present and Functional　　__2__ Present and Not Functional
　　　　　　(21) __3__ Needed and Not Present　Remarks: _____

CHEMICALS: (History of Ingestion)　(22) __N__ None　__P__ Positive　__X__ No Information
　Type:　(23) __1__ Alcohol　(24) __2__ Carbon Monoxide　(25) __3__ Barbiturate　(26) __4__ Tranquilizer
　　　(27) __5__ Amphetamine　(28) __6__ Opiate　(29) __7__ Hallucinogen　(30) __8__ Antihistamine
　　　(31) __9__ Other: (Specify)
Remarks: _____
_____
_____

PSYCHOLOGICAL: (32) __U__ Not Investigated　　__I__ Investigated (Attach Summary)
Remarks: _____

SOCIO-ECONOMIC STATUS: (Family Annual Income)
　(33) __1__ (Less than $3,000)　__2__ ($3,001 to $6,000)　__3__ ($6,001 to $12,000)
　　　__4__ (Greater than $12,000)　__5__ Unknown
Remarks: _____

PHYSICAL FACTORS

POSITION IN VEHICLE: (34) __1__ Driver/Operator　__2__ Passenger　__3__ Pedestrian　__4__ Unknown
　Seat Occupied:　(35) __1__ Front　__2__ Back　__3__ Tailgate　__4__ Seat on Bus
　　　　　　　　__5__ Other: (Specify) _____　　__6__ Unknown
　Position of Tailgate Seat: Facing: (36) __F__ Forward　__R__ Rearward　__C__ Center
Remarks: _____

TYPE OF VEHICLE: (37) __1__ Car　__2__ Station Wagon　__3__ Truck　__4__ Bus
　__5__ Motorcycle　__6__ Motor Scooter　__7__ Tractor-Trailer　__8__ Farm Vehicle
　__9__ Military Vehicle (Other Than Above): _____
　__0__ Other: (Specify) _____
Remarks: (Include No. of wheels, passengers, etc.) _____

MAKE OF VEHICLE: (i.e., Chevrolet, Ford, Dodge, Rambler) (38-45) _____
MODEL OF VEHICLE: (i.e., Impala, Mustang, Dart, Classic) (46-53) _____
YEAR OF VEHICLE: (54-55) 19____　SERIAL NUMBER (56-72) _____

| CASE NO. | AUTOPSY NO. |

FACTORS CONTRIBUTING TO ACCIDENT

PHYSICAL FACTORS (continued)

BODY STYLE: (73) ___1 2-Door with Center Post   ___2 4-Door with Center Post
             ___3 2-Door with No Center Post   ___4 4-Door with No Center Post
             ___5 2-Door with Convertible Top   ___6 4-Door with Convertible Top
             ___7 Station Wagon   ___8 Other:
Remarks: (Include color(s) of Car) _____

TYPE OF ACCIDENT: (Refer to ICDA and enter proper code) (74-78) ____ . ____
Remarks: _____

N

POSITION OF VICTIM AT ACCIDENT SCENE: (10) ___1 Pedestrian   ___2 Remained in Vehicle
  ___3 Ejected from Vehicle-Initial Impact   ___4 Ejected from Vehicle-Secondary Impact
Remarks: _____

VISIBILITY OF CLOTHING: (11) ___L Light   ___M Medium   ___D Dark
Remarks: _____

FIRE FOLLOWING IMPACT? (12) ___Y Yes   ___N No
Remarks: _____

SEAT BELT WORN: (13) ___1 Yes – Secured   ___2 Yes – Belt Failure
    ___3 No – Belt Not Installed   ___4 No – Belt Installed But Not Worn   ___5 Unknown
SHOULDER HARNESS WORN: (14) ___1 Yes – Secured   ___2 Yes – Harness Failure
    ___3 No – Harness Not Installed   ___4 No – Harness Installed But Not Worn   ___5 Unknown
HEADREST: (15) ___1 Defective   ___2 Not Defective   ___3 Not Installed   ___4 Unknown
HELMET WORN: (16) ___1 Not Applicable   ___2 Yes   ___3 No   ___4 Unknown
Remarks (as necessary to explain, clarify or describe any entry above): _____

ENVIRONMENTAL FACTORS

WEATHER CONDITION: (17) ___1 Clear   (18) ___2 Cloudy   (19) ___3 Windy
PRECIPITATION: (20) ___0 None   ___1 Fog   ___2 Rain   ___3 Hail   ___4 Sleet   ___5 Snow
Remarks: _____

ROAD CONDITION: (21) ___1 Dry   (22) ___2 Wet   (23) ___3 Ice   (24) ___4 Snow   (25) ___5 Oil
    (26) ___6 Slush   (27) ___7 Gravel   (28) ___8 Other:
Remarks: _____

GENERAL TIME OF DAY: (29) ___1 Dawn   ___2 Day   ___3 Dusk   ___4 Night
DAY OF WEEK: (30) ___1 Sun   ___2 Mon   ___3 Tue   ___4 Wed   ___5 Thu   ___6 Fri   ___7 Sat
HOLIDAY OR HOLIDAY WEEKEND: (31) ___Y Yes   ___N No

CASE NO.	AUTOPSY NO.

FACTORS CONTRIBUTING TO ACCIDENT

ENVIRONMENTAL FACTORS (continued)

ROAD SURFACE: (32) ___ 1 Cement   ___ 2 Asphalt   ___ 3 Dirt   ___ 4 Other:

TYPE OF HIGHWAY: Limited Access? (33) ___ Y Yes   ___ N No   ___ X Unknown

Total No. of Lanes: (34) ___   Opposite Lanes Separated by Barrier: (35) ___ Y Yes   ___ N No

Remarks:

SECTION OF ROAD: (36) ___ 1 Straight-a-way   (37) ___ 2 Curve Right Angle   (38) ___ 3 Curve Left Angle

(39) ___ 4 Hill Incline   (40) ___ 5 Hill Decline   (41) ___ 6 Intersection

If at Intersection was it (42) ___ C Controlled? or (43) ___ U Uncontrolled?

Type of Control: (44) ___ 1 2-Way Stop   ___ 2 4-Way Stop   ___ 3 Signal

___ 4 Yield   ___ 5 Other:

Remarks: _____

GENERAL LOCATION: (45) ___ B Business (High Population Density)

___ S Suburban/Residential (Low Population Density)   ___ R Rural Area

___ M Military Installation   ___ 0 Other: _____

Remarks: _____

MECHANICAL FACTORS — From Inspection of Vehicle

DOOR LOCKS: (46) ___ 1 Defective   ___ 2 Not Defective and Locked

___ 3 Not Defective and Not Locked   ___ 4 Undetermined   ___ 5 Not Applicable

WINDSHIELD: (47) ___ 1 Broken   ___ 2 Not Broken   ___ 3 Undetermined

STEERING ASSEMBLY: (48) ___ 1 Defective   ___ 2 Not Defective   ___ 3 Undetermined

BRAKES: (49) ___ 1 Defective   ___ 2 Not Defective   ___ 3 Undetermined

HEAD LIGHTS: (50) ___ 1 Defective   ___ 2 Not Defective   ___ 3 Undetermined

TAIL LIGHTS: (51) ___ 1 Defective   ___ 2 Not Defective   ___ 3 Undetermined

BRAKE LIGHTS: (52) ___ 1 Defective   ___ 2 Not Defective   ___ 3 Undetermined

WINDSHIELD WIPERS: (53) ___ 1 Defective   ___ 2 Not Defective   ___ 3 Undetermined

DEFROSTER: (54) ___ 1 Defective   ___ 2 Not defective   ___ 3 Undetermined

HORN: (55) ___ 1 Defective   ___ 2 Not Defective   ___ 3 Undetermined

EXHAUST SYSTEM: (56) ___ 1 Defective   ___ 2 Not Defective   ___ 3 Undetermined

FUEL TANK: (57) ___ 1 Ruptured   ___ 2 Not Ruptured   ___ 3 Undetermined

TIRES: (58) ___ 1 Blowout   ___ 2 Other Defect   ___ 3 Not Defective   ___ 4 Undetermined

INTERIOR SPACE LOST: (59) ___ 0 None   (60) ___ 1 Front   (61) ___ 2 Rear   (62) ___ 3 Top   (63) ___ 4 Unknown

Remarks: (Specify defects indicated above.) _____

_____

_____

_____

_____

_____

_____

_____

_____

| | CASE NO. | | AUTOPSY NO. |

| CASE NO. | | | AUTOPSY NO. |

FACTORS CONTRIBUTING TO ACCIDENT

FAMILIARITY WITH VICINITY OF ACCIDENT

(64) _____ 1 Local Resident _____ 2 Non-Resident _____ 3 Unknown

Remarks: _____
_____
_____
_____
_____
_____

RELATED INFORMATION

PREVIOUS MOVING TRAFFIC VIOLATIONS: (65) _____ Y Yes   _____ N No   __X__ Unknown
(List Violations Below.)

NUMBER OF PEOPLE INJURED IN THIS ACCIDENT: (66-67) _____

Remarks: _____
_____

IDENTITY OF RELATED DEATHS: (Attach additional sheets of paper if necessary.)

	Case No.	Autopsy No.	(Reserved)
Ø	1. (10-19) _____	(20-29) _____	(30-37) _____
P	2. (10-19) _____	(20-29) _____	(30-37) _____
Q	3. (10-19) _____	(20-29) _____	(30-37) _____
R	4. (10-19) _____	(20-29) _____	(30-37) _____
S	5. (10-19) _____	(20-29) _____	(30-37) _____

Remarks: _____
_____
_____
_____

LIST TRAFFIC CONVICTIONS: _____
_____
_____
_____
_____
_____
_____
_____
_____
_____
_____
_____
_____
_____
_____
_____

SUBMITTING ORGANIZATION:

CASE NO. _____ NAME _____

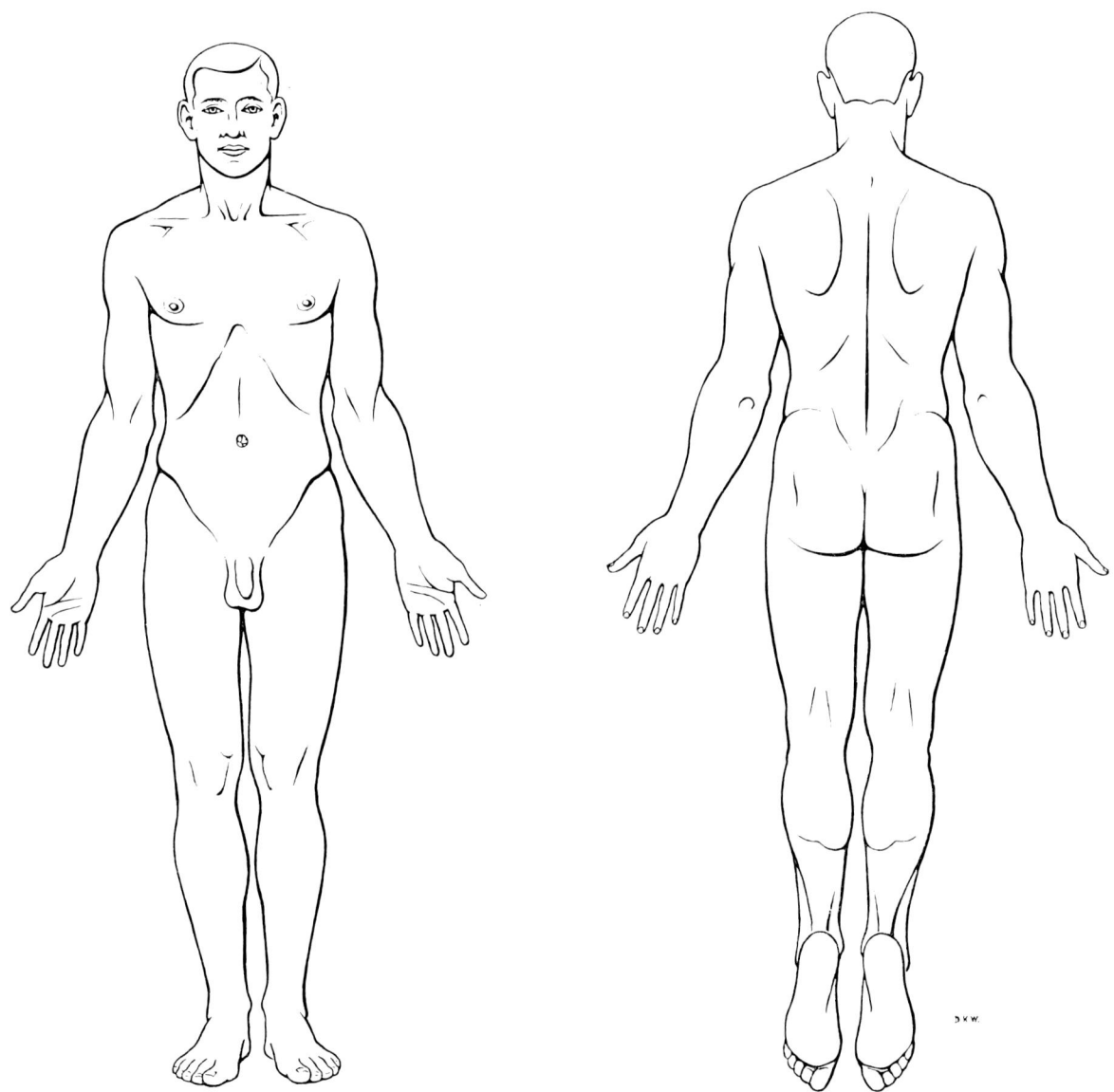

FORM A

CASE NO. _____ NAME _____

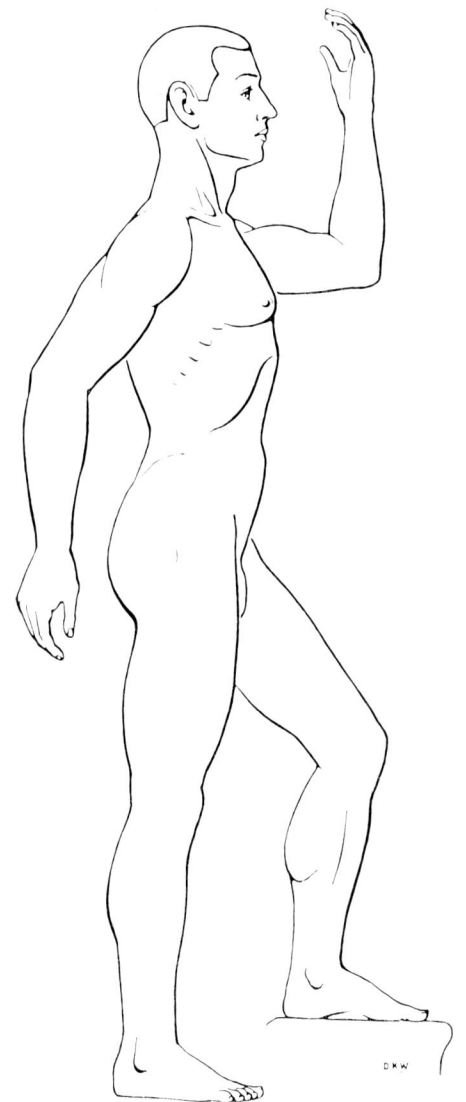 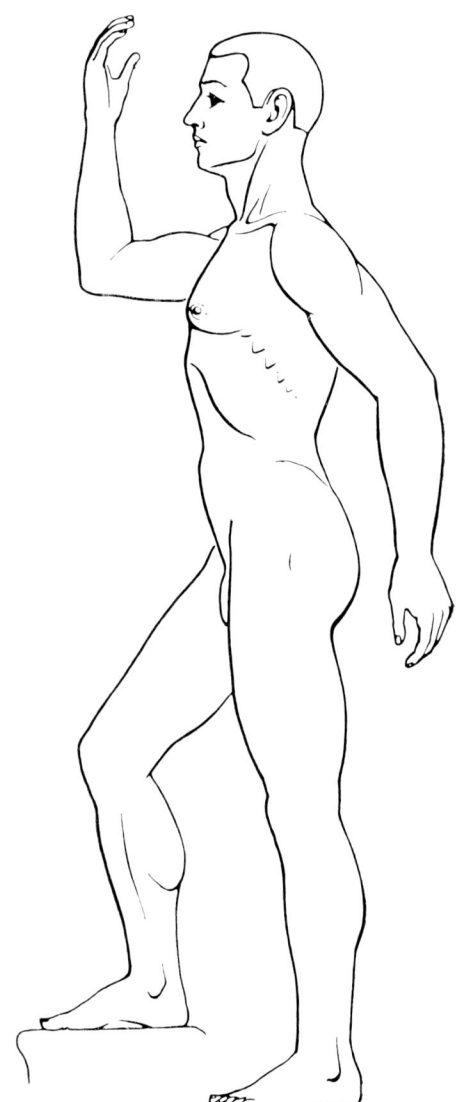

FORM B

Autopsy Information

CASE NO._____ **NAME**_____

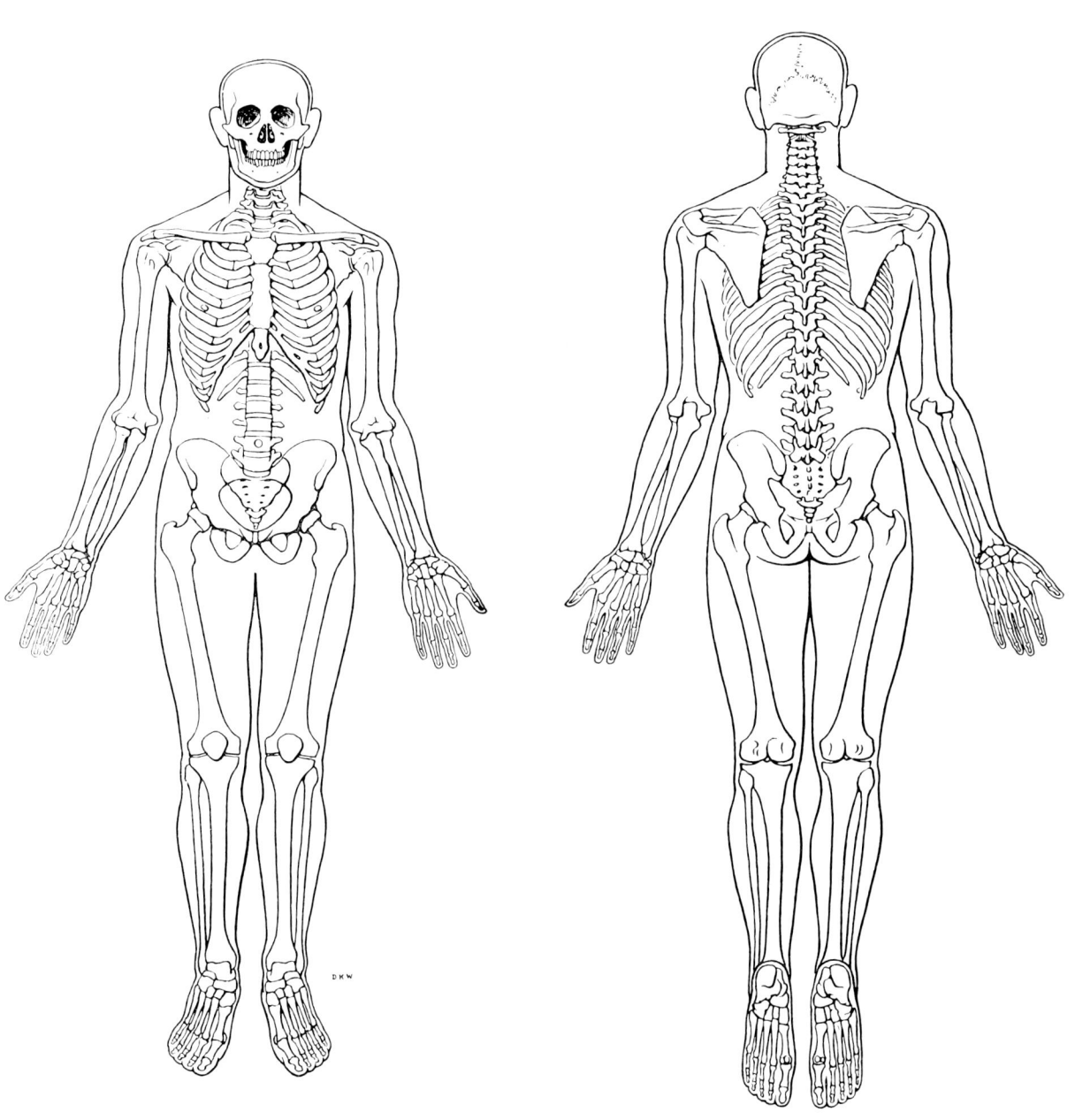

FORM C

CASE NO. _____ **NAME** _____

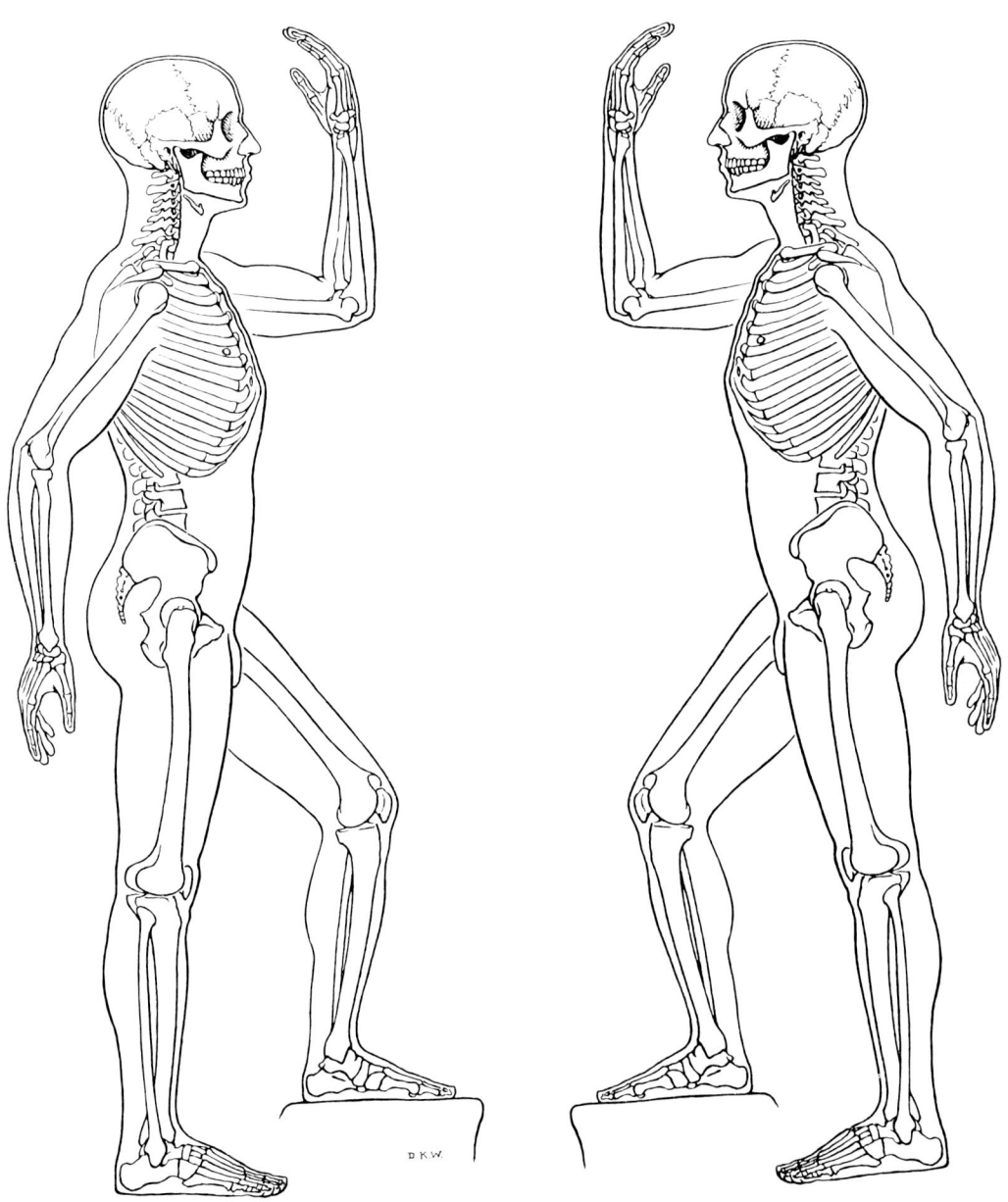

FORM D

CASE NO. _____ **NAME** _____

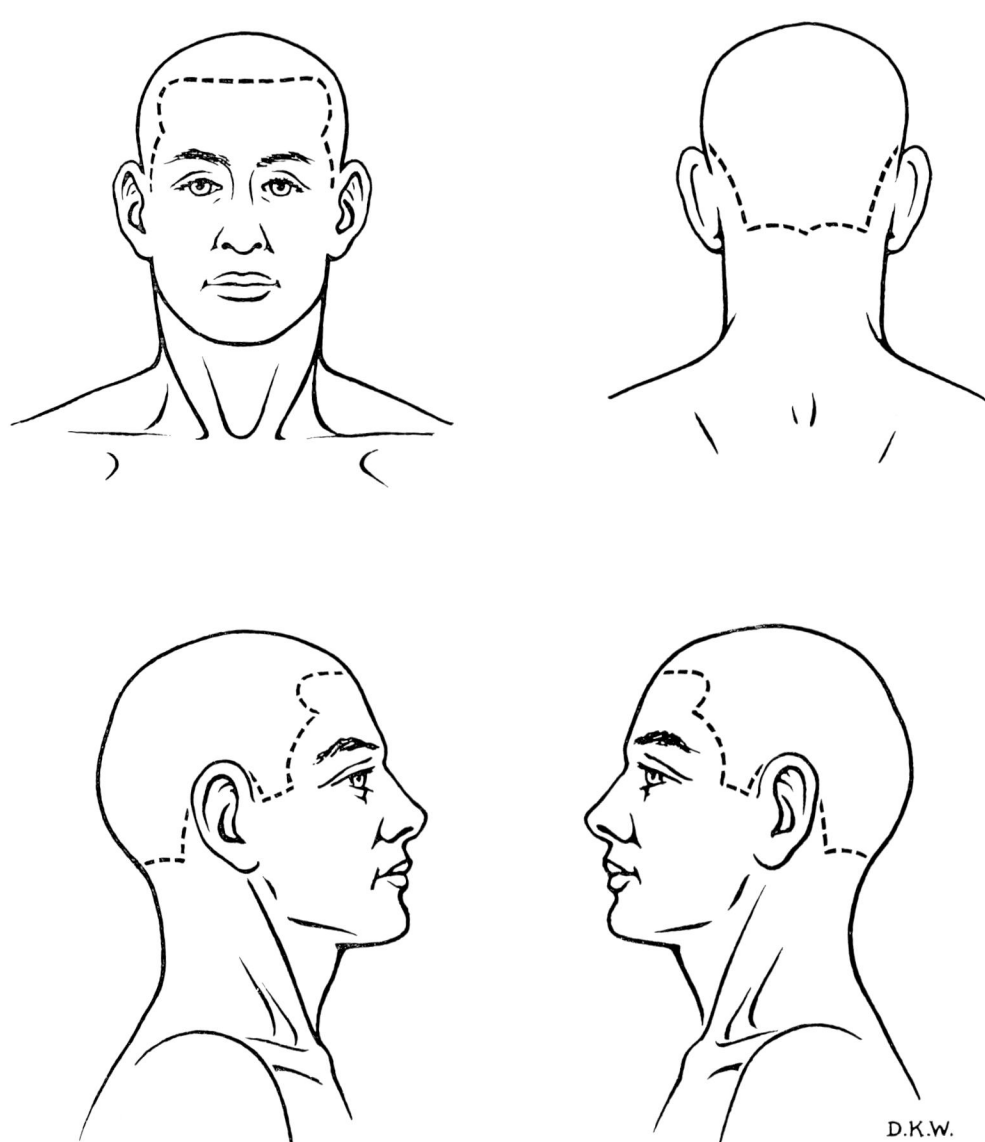

FORM E

CASE NO. _____ NAME _____

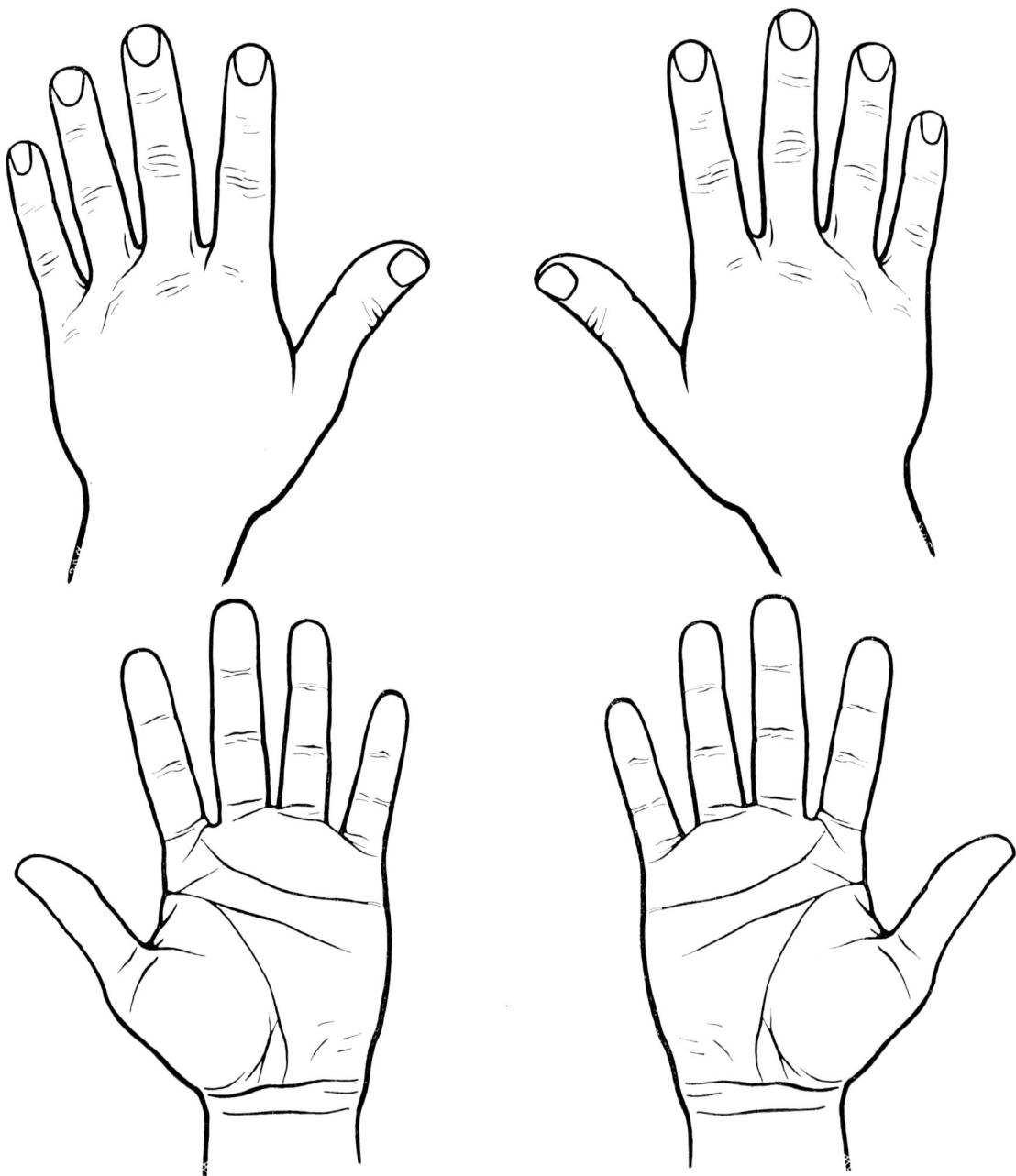

FORM F

Autopsy Information

CASE NO. _____ **NAME** _____

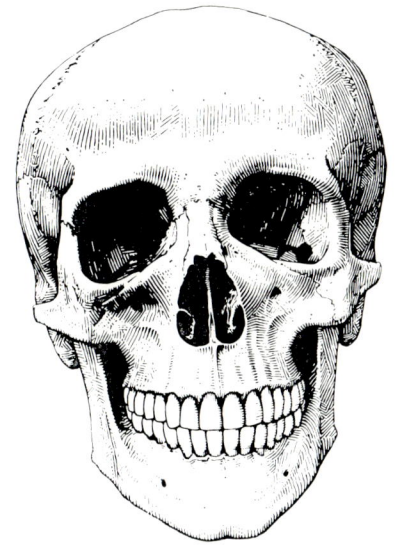
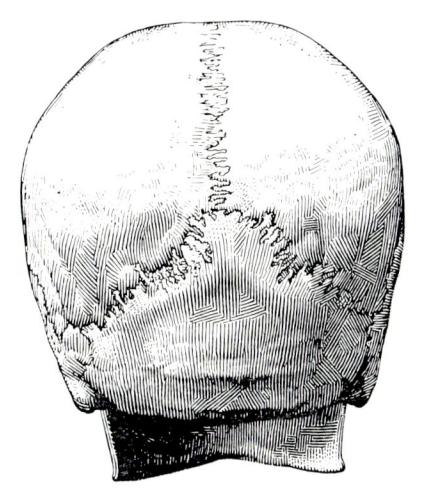
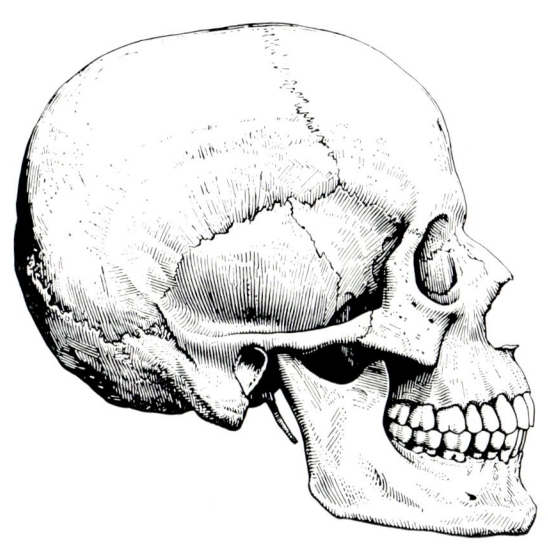
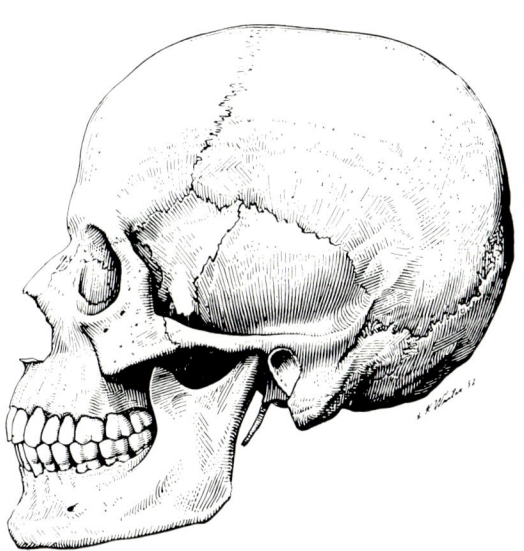

FORM G

CASE NO. _____ NAME _____

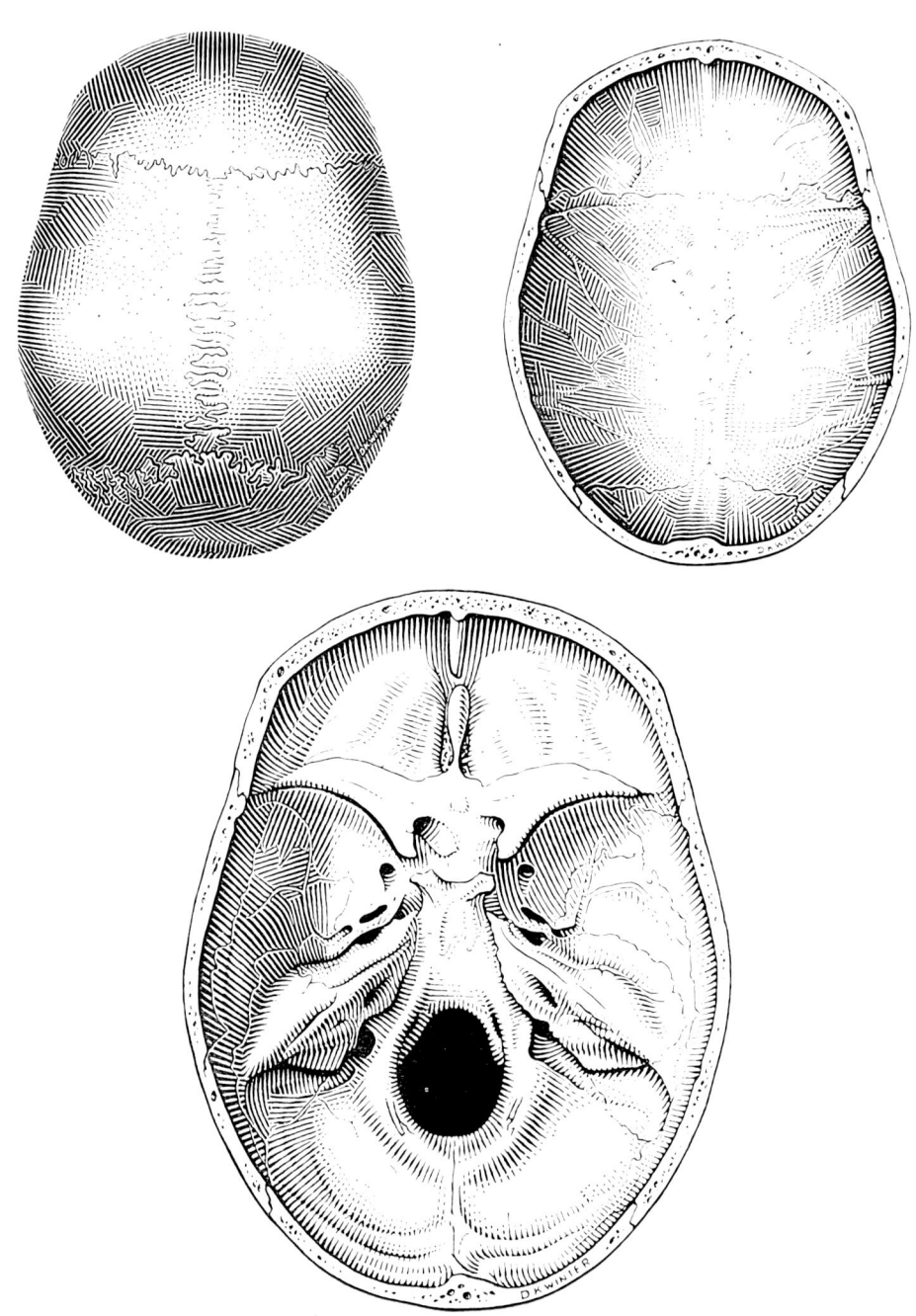

FORM H

CASE NO. _____ NAME _____

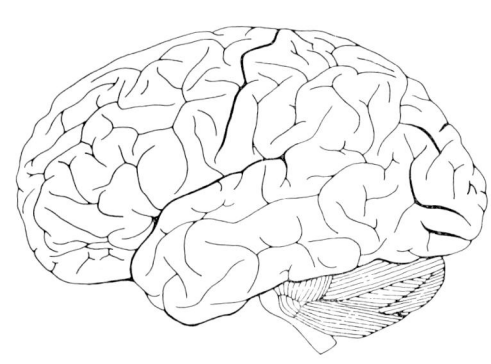

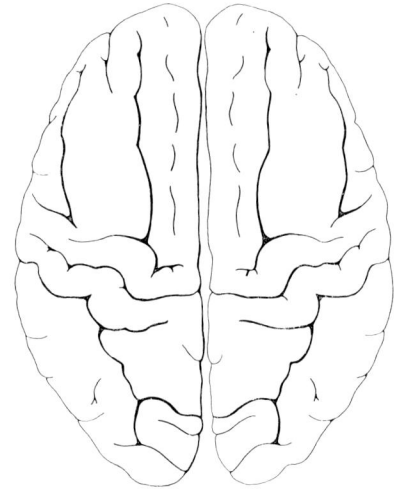

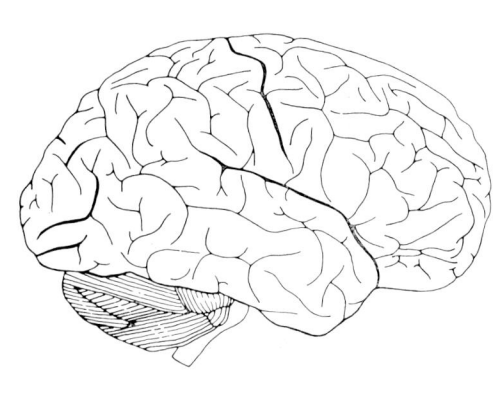

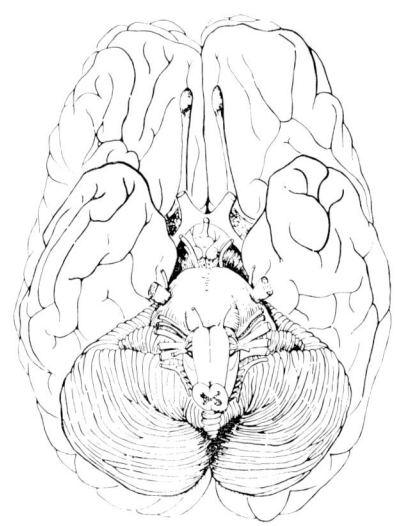

FORM I

CASE NO. _____ NAME _____

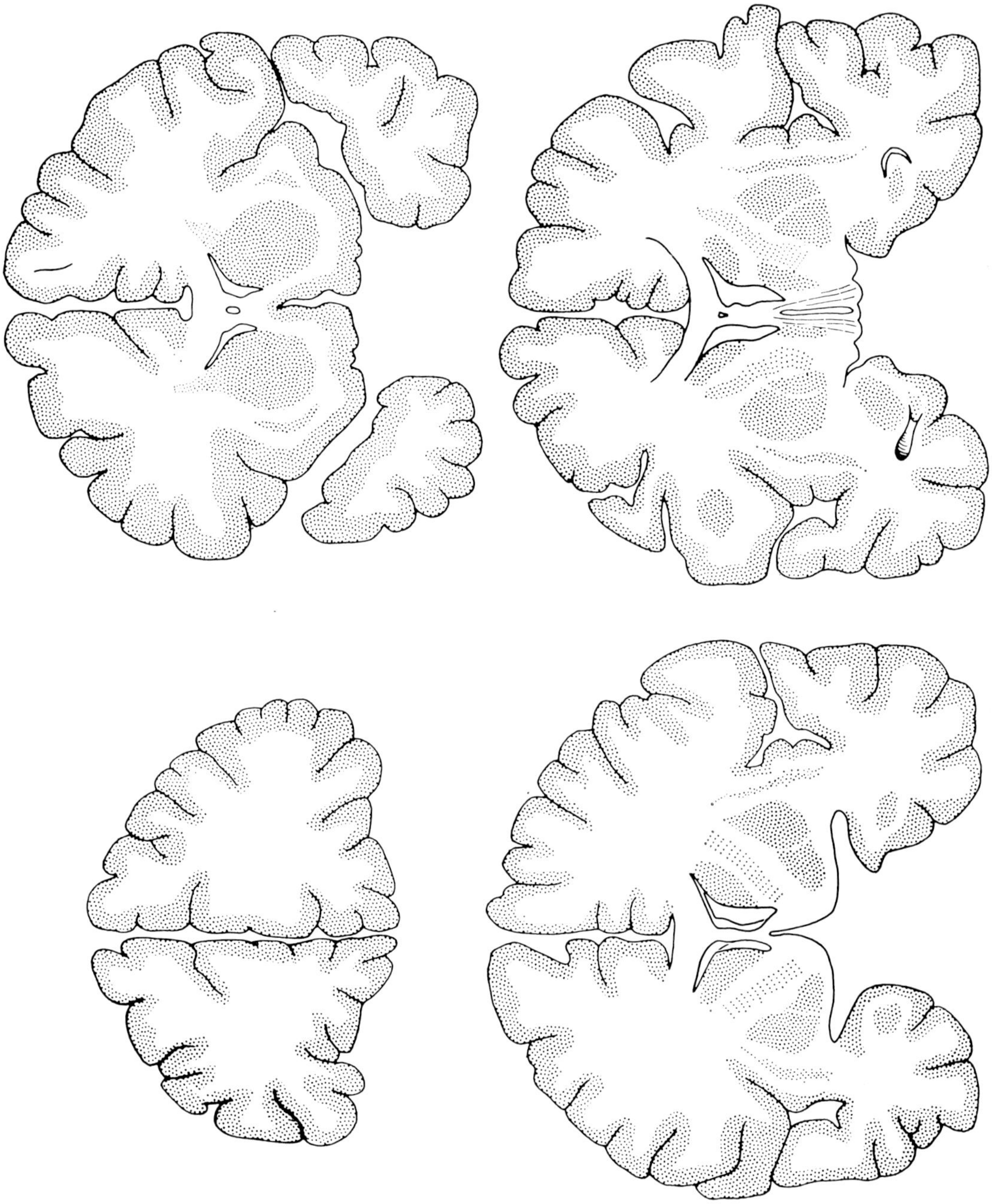

FORM J

Autopsy Information

CASE NO. ———— NAME ————

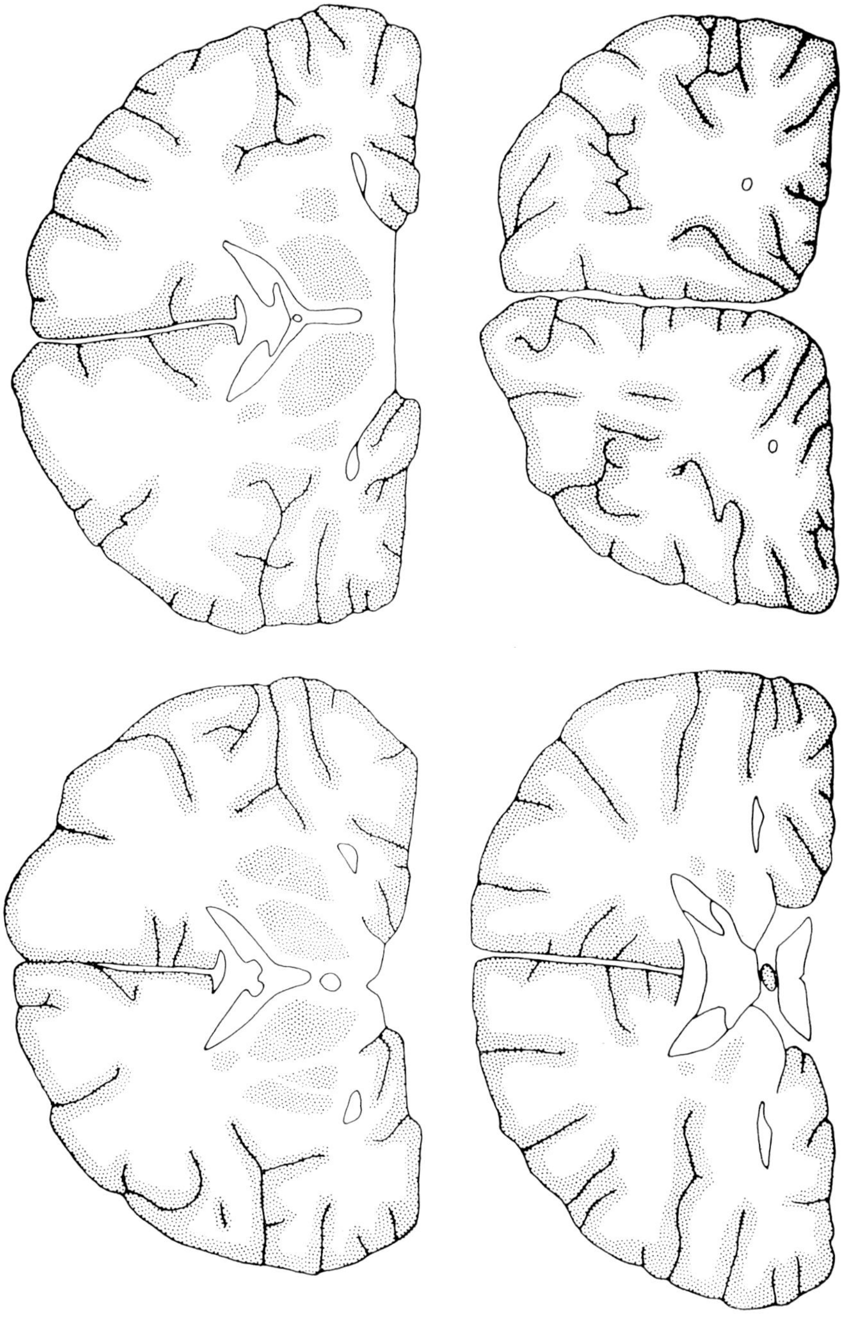

FORM K

CASE NO. _____ NAME _____

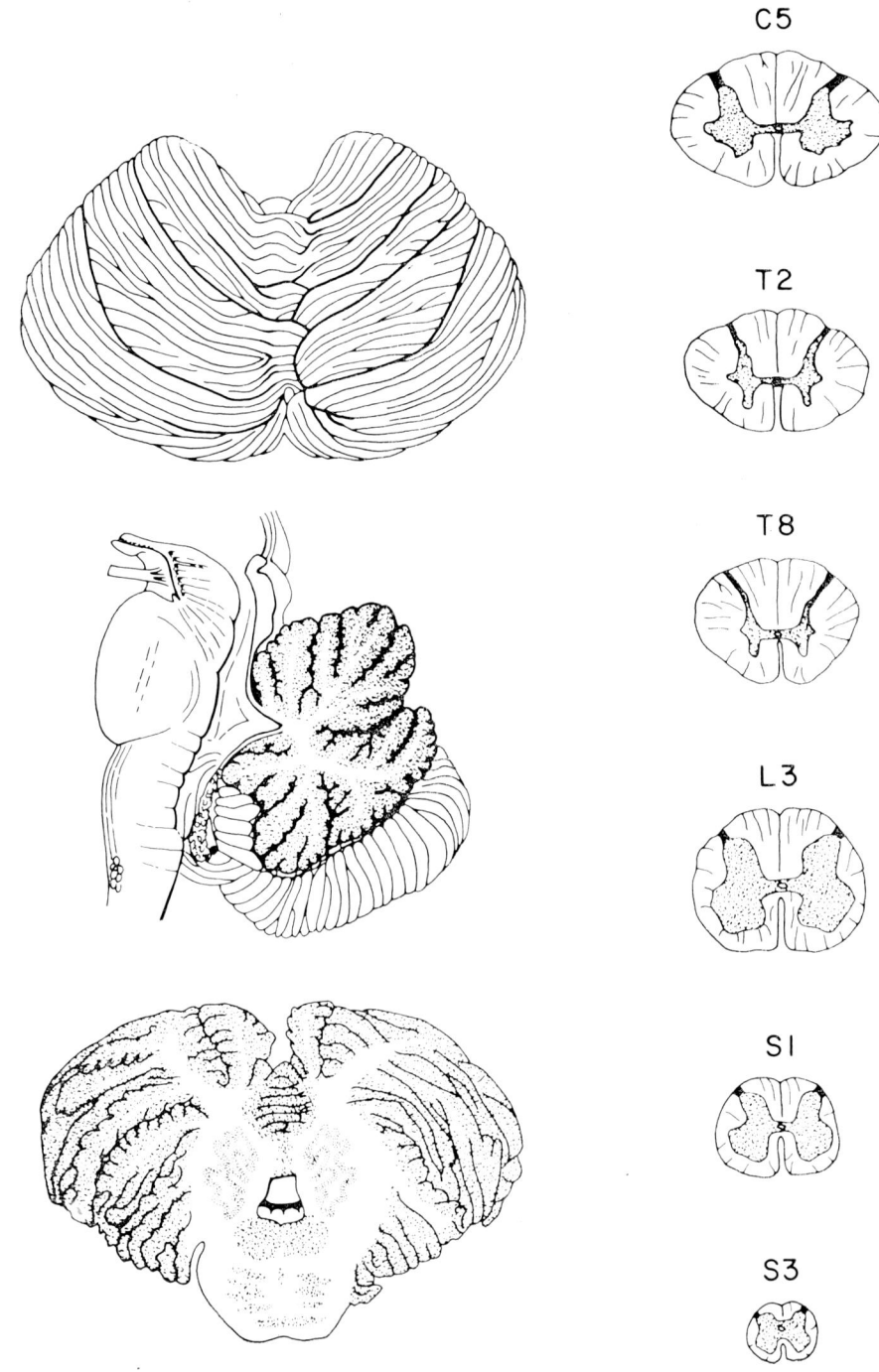

FORM L

CASE NO. _____ NAME _____

RESPIRATORY SYSTEM

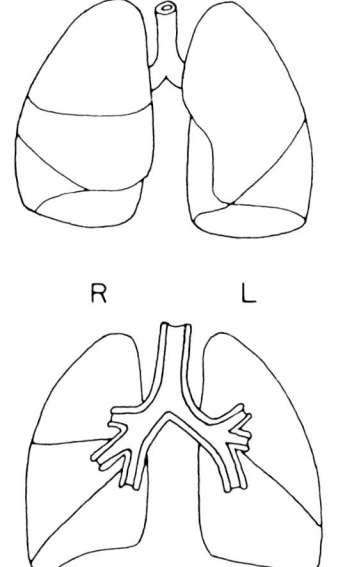

R   L

CARDIOVASCULAR SYSTEM

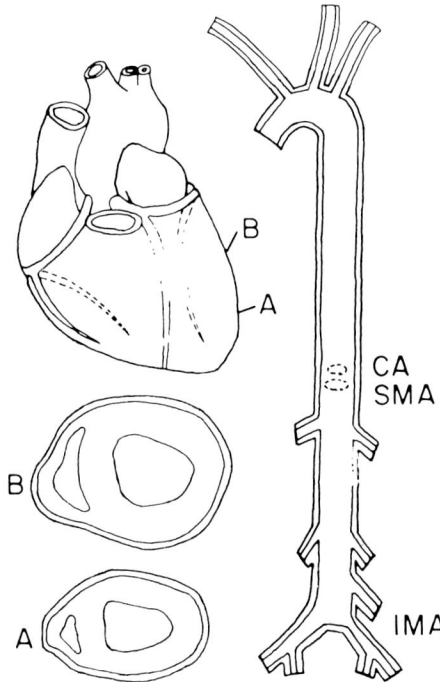

FORM M

CASE NO._____ NAME_____

ALIMENTARY SYSTEM

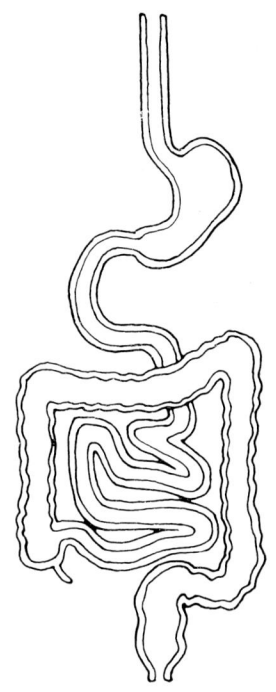

BILIARY SYSTEM

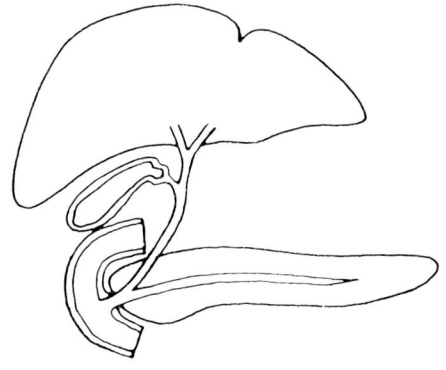

FORM N

CASE NO. _____ NAME _____

HEMATOPOIETIC SYSTEM

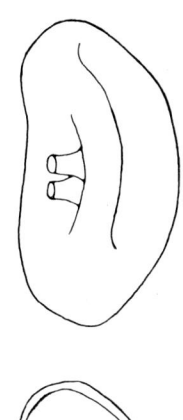

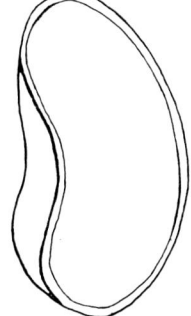

URINARY SYSTEM

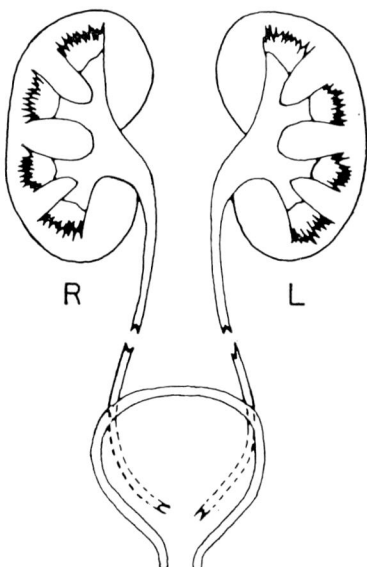

FORM O

CASE NO._____ NAME_____

MALE REPRODUCTIVE SYSTEM

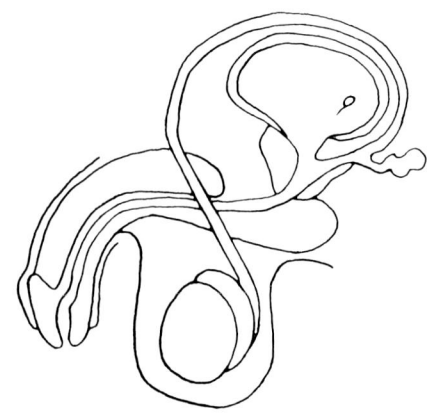

FEMALE REPRODUCTIVE SYSTEM

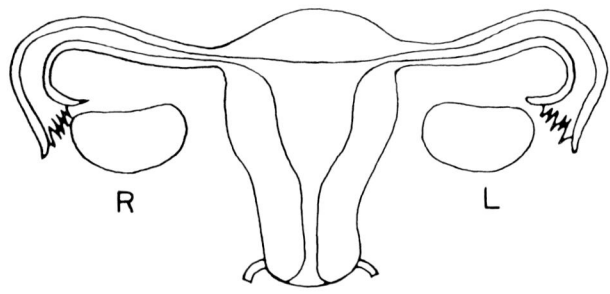

FORM P

CASE NO. _____ NAME _____

ENDOCRINE SYSTEM
Thyroid

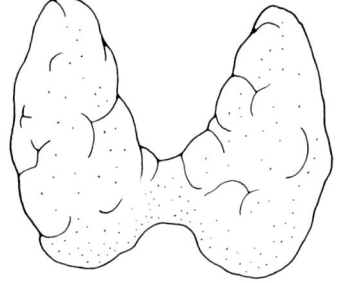

Adrenals

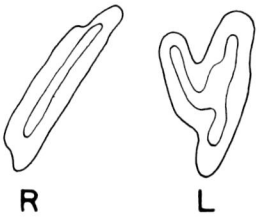

R   L

Pituitary

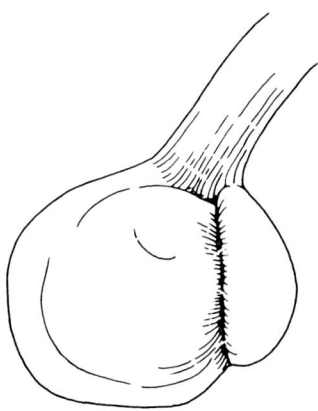

FORM Q

CODING, STORAGE, AND RETRIEVAL OF INFORMATION

With computers in ever greater use today, simple coding systems which allow the reduction of diagnosis to numerical symbols, have been developed. A system widely used is the SNOP or Standard Nomenclature of Pathology. In this system, diagnoses are coded as numbers. Each organ system is assigned a number, and diagnoses corresponding to that system are each given numbers; for example, thymus is coded as 98, thymoma as M8580. This system facilitates both indexing and cross-indexing of information. Computer storage of information is greatly facilitated by the reduction of diagnosis to numbers.

Computer systems can described as both "off-line" and "in-line." An "in-line system" which allows somewhat quicker retrieval of information is the costlier of the two types.

At this hospital an "off-line" system is employed. The patient's name, age, hospital number, and date of hospitalization are typed onto a punch tape along with all coded diagnoses. The punch tapes from all departments of the hospital are placed on a translating system which then places them on magnetic tape. The information may be stored on a magnetic tape or retranslated to a disc for storage. Disc-stored information is quicker to retrieve, requiring only minutes. Magnetic tape stored information is retrieved in a few hours employing an "in-line" system.

UTILIZATION OF THE RESULTS OF AUTOPSY

The literal translation of the Greek "αυτοπσειν" is "to see for oneself." Many autopsies are performed by a pathologist with a desire to have accurate follow-up of interesting or puzzling surgical specimens. However, the most important function of non-medicolegal autopsy is the instruction of clinicians, residents, and, in a university setting, medical students as to the nature of the disease process. This involves demonstration of both gross and microscopic findings.

Most departments of pathology hold regular conferences at which gross material is presented to residents, students, and interested clinicians. Material may be demonstrated in the fresh state within several days if adequately refrigerated.

If adequate refrigeration is not available the tissue may be preserved in several ways. It may initially be fixed in Kaiserling I solution and then kept in Kaiserling III. Alternatively, the tissue may be fixed in 10% buffered formalin for 24 hours and then placed in absolute alcohol which will restore the color. Jores' solution is an acceptable substitute.

If autopsy specimens are to be preserved for prolonged periods, the most reliable method is to seal them in plastic bags. A variety of machines are available which can seal these bags by means of heat. It is also possible to use these heat-sealers to construct bags out of sheets of heavy plastic. Specimens kept in these bags should have a small amount of any of the above-mentioned fixatives included.

For museum demonstration, glass containers sealed by tape or epoxy cement are preferred.

Photography

The most important method of preserving teaching specimens obtained at autopsy is by photography. The optimal state is that in which a professional photographer with all necessary equipment is available at all times. Failing that, alternative methods are available.

Thirty-five mm color film is the most versatile film for the preparation of teaching slides. This is available in rolls of 20 and 36 exposures and as bulk film which may be cut into smaller and larger segments. One advantage of smaller segments is the ease of development without exposing an entire 36 exposure roll.

The camera should be fixed on a stand with a rack and pinion mount for focusing. Preferably, the lens should be a so-called "macro-lens" (50 mm) which allows exposures with a wide angle of vision at close distance. A second choice is a wide-angle lens (35 or 28 mm) which requires extension tubes for close-up views of lesions.

The background is usually blue or green beneath plate glass. The light source may be of several types:

1. The most effective source is stroboscopic lighting from both sides of the specimen. This type of illumination has the advantage of showing no reflection from large reflectors.

2. Secondarily, two tungsten lamps with reflectors may be used, but the reflectors may be seen in the photograph.

3. Movie-type lights may be used, but these have a short life span and are expensive.

If the texture of the specimen is especially important it may be desirable to use only one light or to balance the light to produce a shaded picture.

Some specimens, for example, papillary carcinoma of the bladder and papillary carcinoma of the rectum, are often better photographed underwater, which allows the papillary fronds to float freely. Attention must be paid to prevent reflections from the water surface.

In institutions where few pictures are taken and in cases where charts must be reproduced, Polaroid® units are available for the production of lantern slides. There are also automated cameras which may be used, such as the Kodak Instamatic® line.

Special cameras that have preset frames which are placed against the desired field of view, which are automatically focused, and which have accompanying flash units are available for photography of the cadover (rather than the excised specimen).

In taking a gross photograph there are a few considerations that must be stressed. The specimen should occupy the entire field. The label and the specimen are both to be in focus. There are no unwanted shadows or reflections of the lights.

Photomicrography

Photomicrography is best done by a professional photographer. For our purpose it suffices to state that each microscope and camera be calibrated with the microscope's light source and the type of film by exposing trial rolls of film at different exposures. (See section on fixation and processing of tissue.)

Fixation and Processing of Tissues

The most commonly used fixative for routine autopsy sections is 10% neutral buffered formalin. This is a relatively rapid fixative, and it provides good nuclear detail. It is not necessary to wash formalin-fixed tissue, but a brief washing period may help to remove "formalin pigment" from the tissues.

Some pathologists prefer to use Zenker's solution, a combination of mercuric chloride dichromate and potassium for fixation. We feel that this produces better nuclear staining than formalin, but it has the disadvantages of requiring prolonged washing (at least 24 hours) to remove the chromate pigment and of producing a more brittle specimen which is more difficult to cut. Recently, a modified Zenker's solution using zinc chloride rather than chromium has been described which obviates the necessity of prolonged washing of the specimen, and no precipitated chromium pigment is present.

Another fixative in common use is Bouin's solution. This is a mixture of picric acid, formalin, and acetic acid. This has the advantage of being a very rapid fixative and may be effectively used for the fixation of small specimens. There are, however, very definite disadvantages. The hardening effect of picric acid is so effective that in large blocks the surface may be fixed, prohibiting infiltration of the central portion of the specimen. Also, it is necessary to completely remove all traces of picric acid from the block before processing. It has been stated that retention of picric acid within the block exercises a deleterious effect on the staining of the specimen and that this effect continues over a period of years even within the block.[1]

In fixing specimens where water-soluble substances are to be stained, e.g. glycogen, the best fixatives are either absolute alcohol or Carnoys' solution which is a mixture of absolute alcohol, chloroform, and glacial acetic acid.

If the autopsy is performed soon after death, and autolysis has not occurred and electron microscopic examination is desired, the specimen should be cut into very small fragments and fixed in either osmic acid or gluteraldehyde. It is imperative that these specimens be submitted as very small (less than 0.1 cm) fragments for rapid and adequate fixation. It is possible to make adequate electron micrographs on formalin-fixed tissue, but the best sections are made from sections fixed immediately in gluteraldehyde. The most important factor is the time expended between the death of the patient and the removal of the specimen. The fine structure of any organ or cell is best appreciated when that time space is minimized.

One important facet of processing tissue is decalfication. Several methods are available: dilute (5%) nitric acid, a buffered 10% formic acid, 20% sodium citrate solution, and commercial "rapid decal" solutions may be used. There are also electrolytic decalcification apparatuses available. In the chemical decalcifying methods it is important to observe two points. The specimen must be thoroughly washed after decalcification. The specimen must be tested for completeness of decalcification at frequent intervals. This second part applies also to electrolytic decalcification methods. Over-decalcification is tantamount to "overkill." All of these procedures damage the appearance of cells in the final histopathologic slide.

The processing of tissue for sectioning is essentially a sequence of dehydration and infiltration with formalin. Most laboratories use automated machines for this purpose, and the reader is directed for further information about specific staining and special processing to several books devoted to that subject.[1-4]

REFERENCES

1. Luna, Lee G. (Ed.): *Manual of Histologic Staining Methods of the Armed Forces Institute of Pathology*, 3rd ed. McGraw-Hill, New York, 1968.
2. Barka, T., and Anderson, P. J.: *Histochemistry; Theory, Practice and Bibliography.* Harper & Row, New York, 1963.
3. Lillie, R. D.: *Histopathologic Technic and Practical Histochemistry*, 3rd ed. McGraw-Hill, New York, 1965.
4. Pearse, A. G. E.: *Histochemistry; Theoretical and Applied*, 2nd ed. Little, Brown, Boston, 1960.

Appendix

ORGAN WEIGHTS

It is difficult to give the exact weight of various organs without preparing large tables of weights, because many organs vary with both the weight of the adult body and also the age of the patient.

A few rough weights should be included for the adult standard male of 40 kg.

Heart: 300-350 gm.

This will vary between 250-400 gm depending on the weight of the patient.

Lungs: 250 gm each.

In most autopsies because of severe congestion, these weights will be increased.

Liver: 1300 gm

Spleen: 150 gm

Pancreas: Up to 100 gm

Adrenals: 15 gm combined.

Kidneys: 150-200 gm each.

Thyroid: Up to 40 gm

INDEX

A
Abdomen, 5
Abdominal cavity, 16-18, 21-24 figs., 28-29, 68
Abnormalities, 40-41, 68
Abortion, 8
Accident pathology, 71-74
    aquatic accidents, 73-74
    automobile accidents, 71-73
    electrical accidents, 74
    home accidents, 73
    medicolegal autopsy, 71
Acute pulmonary emphysema, 74
Acute subdural hematoma, 8
Adrenal glands, 29, 38
    weight, 115
Aggravated misdemeanor, 3
Air emboli
    aquatic accidents, 74
    detection of, 67
Alcohol fixative, 113-14
Alcoholism, 3, 8
Amyloid testing, 11
Anesthetic procedure, death from, 8
Aneurysm, 60
Anus, 29
Aorta, 18
Appendix, 38
Aquatic accidents, 73-74
Arson, 8
Assault, 8
    body of decedent, 3
Aunts, 3
Automobile accidents, 71-73
    form for recording data, 72
Autopsy room, 10-12
    access to, 10
    adjustable height of table, 10-11 fig.
    air conditioning, 10
    attendant's preparation of, 13
    automobile accident victim, inspection and treatment of, 72
    band-saw, 12
    blade sharpener, 12
    bone forceps, 41
    bottles, 12
    brain cutting board, 62
    buckets, 12
    cabinet for supplies, 10
    chisels, 12, 41
    clothing available for, 10
    copper solutions, 11
    dictaphone recording, 75
    dictating apparatus, 12
    dissecting instruments, 12 fig.
    dissecting room lighting, 10
    dissecting table with ventilating equipment, 11
    dressing room adjacent to, 10
    electrically-powered vibrating saw, 12, 41
    enterotome, 12
    equipment, 10-12
        organ review conferences, 11-12
    fixatives, 12
    floor covering, 10
    fluid measuring receptacle, 10
    forceps, 12, 41
    form filled out in, 75
    formalin jars and buckets, 10-11
    hammers, 12, 41
    heat sealing iron for plastic bags, 13 fig.
    instruments
        cleanliness of, 14
        dissecting, 12 fig.
        nervous system, 41
    iodine solutions, 11
    Jores' solution for preservation, 11, 75
    knives, 11-12, 41
    labeling of jars and buckets, 11
    lighting, 10
    location, 10
    marking of, 10
    ozone purifiers, 10
    probes, 12
    procedures following autopsy in, 75-76
    refrigerators, 11
    scales, small and large, 11
    scissors, 12, 41
    shower, 10
    sink drain, 10
    smaller bottles for sections, 10-11
    soap, availability and type of, 10
    sponge availability, 14
    supplies, 10-12
        organ review conferences, 11-12
    table placement, size, shape and number, 10
    table tilt and suction apparatus, 10-11 fig.
    uniform for pathologist, 10
    ventilation, 10
    vibrating electric saw, 12, 41
    wall paint, 10
    water supply, 10
    wide-mouthed jars for formalin or Zenker's solution, 10
    window requirements, 10
    working conditions required, 10
    yardstick, 11

B
Bacterial poisoning, 8
"Baseball" stitch for incisions, 8
Biblical injunction, 5
Biliary tree, 34
Bladder, 26, 29, 39
Blood
    cleansing off, 8
    distribution at scene of automobile accident, 72
    typing, 72
Body temperature, 71, 73
Bone evaluation, 26
Bouin's solution, 113
Boyle, law of, 67, 74
Brain, 29
    anatomical distortions, reasons for and avoidance of, 44
    cutting board for, 62
    definitive gross examination, 60-66 figs.
    fixation, 51-52
    lethal intracerebral lesion, 52
    massive subarachnoid hemorrhage, 51
    microscopic examination, 64
    removal, 47-51 figs.
    sectioning procedure, 62-66
    slicing procedure, 62-66
Brainstem, 61 fig., 62-63 fig., 65 fig.
Breasts, 15, 17 figs.
Burial permit, 8
Burns from electrocution, 74

C
Cadaver, care of, 8-9
Calvarium, 44-47 figs.
    elderly persons, 47
    infancy, 47

Cameras for photographing specimens, 113
Carnoys' solution, 113-14
Cerebellum, 62-63 fig., 64-65 fig.
Cerebrum, 62 fig., 65 fig.
Cervical pedicles, 56-57 figs.
Chest cavity and organs, 18, 24, 29, 68
Chlorides, examination for, 73
Cisterna chyli, 68
Cleanliness of body, 8
Clinical history, reading and knowledge of, 12-13
Clinical record review, 40
Clivus, 53
Coding of information, 112
Colon, 17-18, 23, 38
Common law marriages, 5
Common law spouse, 5
Coma, death following, 8
Computerization of information, 112
Consent for autopsy, 3-5
  common law spouse, 5
  contents, 3-5
  failure to obtain, 3
  form, 4 fig.
  friend in absence of relations, 3
  hospital administrator's approval, 5
  nearest relation, 3
  review of, 12
  sequence of relationship for, 3
  signature of legal next of kin, 12
  telegram, 5
  telephone, 5
  waiting period after, 3
  witness to, 5
  written, 3, 5
Conservative Judaism, 5
Consultations, 40
Contusions, recording of, 40
Convulsive seizure, 8
Coronary arteries, 33
Coroner's order for autopsy, 3
Councilman's chisel, 41
Cousins, 3
Cranial nerves, 51
Cutis anserina, 73
Cysts, 39, 68

D

Death
  cause of, 5-7
  estimation of time of, 70
Death certificate, 5-7
  cause of death, 5-7
  completion of, 8
  contents, 5-7
  form, 6
  purpose, 5
  signature requirement, 7
  signing of, time for, 6
  submission by physician, time for, 6

Decalcification, 114
Decomposed bodies, autopsies on, 69-70
Dental chart recording, 14
Diaphragm, 23-24, 28
Diatoms in lungs, 73
Dictaphone recording, 75
Dictated protocol, 76-78
Discrepancies in names of deceased and next of kin, 13
Diseases, report to local health authorities of, 7
Disposition of unclaimed body to institution, 3
Dissections of individual organs, 29-39 (*see also specific organs*)
Diverticula, 38
Drownings, 73
Drug abuse, 3
Dura, 47-48 fig., 52 fig., 58-61 fig., 64
Dural sinuses, 52-53

E

Ectopic pregnancies, 39
Electrical accidents, 74
Electrocution, 74
Electrolytic decalcification apparatuses, 114
Electron microscopic examination, 114
Embalmed bodies, autopsies on, 69
Embalming process
  facilitation of, 8
  space provided for, 8
Emboli, 26 (*see also* Air emboli)
Endometriosis, 39
Epicardium, 33
Esophageal varices (*see* Esophagus)
Esophagus, 18, 24-25 fig., 29, 34, 36-38, 67
Ethnic considerations, 5
Evisceration
  en bloc, 28-29
  Rokitansky method, 28-29
  Virchow method, 18-28
External examination, 13-14
  nervous system, 40-41
Extremities, 5
  tying of arteries, 8
Eyes, 5, 40-41, 55

F

Fallopian tubes, 29, 39
Fat necrosis testing, 11
Felony, 3
Female genital tract, 39 (*see also specific organs*)
Final anatomic diagnosis (F.A.D.), 75-76
Fingerprints
  automobile accident victim, 72
  body of deceased, 14

Fixation
  autopsy tissues, 113-14
  brain, 51-52
  spinal cord, 59
Forensic autopsy, 71
  purpose, 71
Forensic pathologist, 71
Formalin
  fixative for autopsy specimens, 113
  jars and buckets for, 10-11
Forms
  consent for autopsy, 4
  death certificate, 6
  dictated protocol, 77-78
  physician's medical report, 7
  pictorial protocol, 78-111
Fresh water drowning, 73
Friends, 3
Function of autopsy, 112
Fundamentalist groups, 5
Funeral director
  burial permit, need for, 8
  rapport with pathologist, 8
  release of body to, 8-9

G

Gallbladder, 22, 24, 29, 35 fig.
Gastrointestinal tract, 34-38 figs. (*see also specific organs*)
General considerations, 3-9
General pathologist (*see* Pathologist)
Genital tract, 68 (*see also specific organs*)
Genitourinary tract, 38-39 (*see also specific organs*)
Getler method of analysis for chlorides, 73
Gluteraldehyde, 114
Glycogen, 113
Grandparents, 3
Gross organ review, 9

H

Head, 5, 41-55 (*see also specific parts*)
  measurement of circumference, 40
  newborn autopsy, 67
  tying of arteries, 8
Heart, 22 fig., 33-34
  air emboli, detection of, 67
  weight, 115
Height of patient, 75
Hemorrhage areas, 39
Hemorrhoids, 38
Henry's law, 74
High voltage current, electrocution from, 74
Home accidents, 73
Homicide, 7
Hospital autopsy
  medicolegal autopsy distinguished, 71

Index

Hospitals (*see also* Non-teaching institutions; Teaching institutions)
  time for autopsies, 13
Hyoid bone, 30

I

Illustrations
  anterior bone, 44
  autopsy table, 11
  brain, 50
  brain slice undercutting, 66
  brainstem, 61, 63, 65
  breasts, 17
  calvarium, 45-46
  cerebellum, 65
  cerebrum, 62-63, 65
  cervical pedicles, 57
  dura, 48, 52, 61
  esophagus, 25
  gallbladder, 35
  gastrointestinal block, 35
  globe and optic nerve, 55
  heart, 22
  heat sealing iron for plastic bags, 13
  instruments for dissection, 12
  intestine, 25
  kidney, 27
  liver, 24, 36
  lungs, 23, 31-32
  neck block, 19
  oculomotor nerve, 49
  opening of body, 15-16
  optic nerve, 48, 55
  orbital roof, 54
  pancreatic duct, 35
  pelvic block, 28
  pericardium, 20-21
  petrous bone, 54
  pituitary stalk, 49
  posterior bone, 45
  pulmonary artery, 21
  renal vessels, 26
  scalp, 42
  spinal column, 58
  spinal cord, 59
  spleen, 23, 37
  stomach, 25
  temporalis and temporal bone, 43
  tentorium cerebelli, 50
  thoracic pedicles, 57
  Vena Cava, 22
  Virchow chisel to open vault, 46
Incisions (*see also specific type or area*)
  "baseball" stitch, 8
Individual organ dissections, 29-39 (*see also specific organs*)
Infants' calvarium opening, 47
Information requirements, 75-114
  consent for autopsy, 3-5
  death certificate, 5-7
  toe tag, 13

Injury, death due to, 8
In-line computer system, 112
Inspection of body, 13-14
Instruments
  cleanliness, 14
  dissecting, 12 fig.
  nervous system, 41
Internal examination by Virchow method, 15-18
Intestines, 16-18, 23-25 fig., 38 (*see also* Colon)
Intoxication, 72
Intracranial contents, 41-55 (*see also specific parts*)

J

Jewish denominations, 5
Jores' solution in buckets, 11, 75
Jurisdiction of medical examiner (*see* Medical examiner)

K

Kidneys, 25-27 fig., 29, 38-39
  weight, 115

L

Lacerations, recording of, 40
Large intestine (*see* Colon)
Left atrial appendage, 34
Lesions, 72-73
Lightning, death from, 74
Liver, 22-24 figs., 29, 36 fig.
  weight, 115
Liver mortis, 69-71, 73
Lobectomy cases, 32
Local law governing, 3, 5, 7
  common law marriages, 5
Low voltage current, electrocution from, 74
Lungs, 30-32 figs.
  diatoms in, 73
  weight, 115

M

Magnetic tape stored information, 112
Male genital tract, 39 (*see also specific organs*)
Marrow evaluation, 26
Meckel's diverticulum, 38
Medical examiner
  jurisdiction of, 7-8
    pathologist finding of case within, 8
    relinquishment of, 8
    retention of, 8
  order for autopsy, 3
Medical examiner's cases
  consent, time to secure, 3
  death certificate signature, 7
  military personnel, 3
Medical report, 7

Medicolegal autopsy, 71
  hospital autopsy distinguished, 71
  report, 78-111
Medicolegal problems, absence of, 12
Mesenteric vessels, 16-17, 29
Metastases, 38
Methods of performing autopsy, 10-39 (*see also specific topics*)
Microscopic examinations
  brain, 64
  spinal cord, 65-66
Military personnel, 3
Mongoloid facies, 68
Mouth, 18
Mummification, 70
Muscle, 60
Muscle sections, 26
Museum demonstrations, 112

N

Neck block, 18-19 fig.
Negligence, 8
Neonatal autopsy, 68
Nerve sections, 26
Nerves, 60
Nervous system, 40-66 (*see also specific parts of system*)
  brain, 60-66
  clinical record review, 40
  difficulties encountered, reasons for, 40
  external examination, 40-41
  goal to be achieved, 40
  head contents, 41-55
  instruments, 41
  intracranial contents, 41-55
  music, 60
  nerve, 60
  spinal cord, 55, 60-66
Neurologic autopsy, 40-66 (*see also* Nervous system)
Neurologists, communication with, 40
Neurosurgeons, communication with, 40
Newborn autopsy, 68
New York City
  death certificate form, 6
  jurisdiction of medical examiner, 7-8
  unclaimed bodies, release of, 3
New York City Municipal Hospitals
  consent form for autopsy, 4 fig., 5
Nitrogen narcosis, 74
Non-teaching institutions
  return of organs to body, 9
Nurse's notes, 12-13

O

Occlusive vascular disease, 60
Off-line computer system, 112
Opening the body, 14-16 figs.
Optic nerves, 47-48 figs., 53, 55 fig.

Oral structures, 28
Orbital fat, 55
Orbital roof, 53-55 figs.
Organ review conferences, 75
  supplies and equipment for, 11-12
Organ section cutting for processing, 75
Organ weights, 115
  prosecutor's check for, 75
Orthodox Judaism, 5
Osmic acid, 114
Ovaries, 29
Over-decalcification, 114

P

Palpation
  body, 13-14
  skull, 40
Pancreas, 24, 29, 35 fig.
  weight, 115
Pancreatitis, 11
Parasellar tissue, 53
Parathyroids, 18
Parents, 3
Pathologist
  amended death certificate, 6
  automobile accident autopsy procedure, 71
  clinical history, reading and knowledge of, 12-13
  death certificate signature, 7
  doubt as to jurisdiction, 8
  dressing room for, 10
  embalmed body autopsy, notes on, 69
  finding of case within jurisdiction of medical examiner, 8
  funeral director, working relationship with, 8
  rapport with funeral director, steps for, 8-9
  trauma-caused death, function in, 71
  uniform for, 10
Peculiar deaths, 8
Pelvic block, 28 fig., 29
Pelvic orgns, 23, 26
Penis, 29
Performance of postmortem examination, delay in, 6
Pericardium, 18, 20-21 figs., 67
Peripheral nerves, 60
Permission for autopsy (see Consent for autopsy)
Petrous bone, 53-54 fig.
Pharyngeal structures, 28
Photographs
  automobile accident scene, 72
  automobile accident victim, 72
  autopsy findings, 75
  preservation of autopsy specimens, 112-13

Photomicrography for preservation of autopsy specimens, 113
Physicians
  confidential medical report, 7
  prosecutor's discussion of case with, 13
  submission of death certificate, 6
Picric acid, 113
Pictorial protocol, 76-111
  forensic use, 76
  hospital use, 76
Pituitary gland, 53
Placenta, 68
Plastic bags
  heat sealing iron for, 13 fig.
  organs returned in, 9
Pleura, 18
Poisoning, 8
Polyps, 38
Posterior mitral block, 34
Posterior superior interventricular septum, 34
Postmortem changes, 69-70
Potter's facies, 68
Preliminary incision, 14
Preliminary steps, 13
Preparation for performance of autopsy, 12-13
Preservation methods for specimens, 112-13
Procedures following autopsy, 75-76
Procedures of performing autopsy, 10-39 (see also specific topics)
Processing of autopsy tissues, 113-14
  sectioning purposes, 114
Prosecutor
  discussion of case with physician, 13
  medicolegal problems, absence of, 12
  organ weights, check for, 75
  slides, inspection of and comments on, 75
  toe bag on body, checking of, 13
Prostate, 26, 39
Protestant denominations, 5
Protocols, 76-111
  dictated, 76-78
  pictorial, 76
    forensic use, 76
    hospital use, 76
  verbal, 76-78
Pulmonary arteries, 33
Pulmonary veins, 18, 20-21 figs.
Putrefaction, 70

R

Racial considerations, 5
Rectum, 26, 28
Reformed Judaism, 5
Relations
  absence of, 3, 6
  consent for autopsy, 3
  delay in finding, 6

  more than one of proper degree, 3
  one of several in group, 3
  search for, 3
  sequence for consent for autopsy, 3
  several, 3
Release of body, 8-9
  cleanliness, 8
  identification, 8
Release of remains, 5
Religious considerations, 5
Renal arteries, 25-26 fig., 29
Respiratory tract, 18
Restrictions, 5
Results of autopsy, utilization of, 112-14
Retention of organs for review, 8-9
Retention of tissue for diagnosis, 5
Retina, 55
Retrieval of information, 112
Rib cage, 15, 18, 67
Ribs, 18
Rigor mortis, 69-71, 73
Rinsing of body, 14
Rokitansky method, 28-29
  advantage of, 28
Roman Catholics, 5
Room for autopsy (see Autopsy room)

S

Salt water drowning, 73
Scalp, reflection of, 41-43 figs.
Scars, recording of, 40
Scuba diving equipment failure, 67, 73-74
Search for relations, 3
Sella turcica, 53
Seminal vesicles, 39
Siblings, 3
  children of, 3
Skeletal muscle, 60
Skin, freeing of, 15, 67
Skull
  base, 52-53
  palpation, 40
Slides, inspection and description of, 75
Small intestine, 38
Special procedures, 67-70
  air emboli, detection of, 67
  decomposed bodies, 69-70
  embalmed bodies, 69
  esophagus, 67
  neonatal autopsy, 68
  postmorem changes, 69-70
  thoracic duct, 68
Spinal axis, 41
Spinal cord, 55-60 figs. (see also Vertebral column)
  definitive gross examination, 64-66 figs.
  fixation, 59
  microscopic examination, 65-66

Index

Spleen, 22-23 fig., 36-37 fig.
   weight, 115
Standard Nomenclature of Pathology (SNOP), 112
Stomach, 24-25 fig., 29, 34
Storage of information, 112
Stryker autopsy saw, 41
Suicide, 3, 8
Surgical incisions, noting and describing of, 14, 40
Surgical procedures, death from, 8
Surviving children, 3
Surviving spouse, 3
Suspected homicide, 3
Suspicious origin of death, 3

T
Teaching institutions
   organ review conferences, 75
   retention of organs for review, 8-9
   time for autopsies, 13
Telegram consents, 5
Telephone consents, 5
Tentorium cerebelli, 49-50 fig., 51
Testes, 26, 29, 39
Thoracic cavity, 18, 29
Thoracic duct, 68
Thorax, 5
Thymus, 18, 32
Thyroid, 18, 30
   weight, 115
Time for performance of autopsy, 13
Time for signing death certificate, 6
Time of death, estimation of, 70

Toe tag
   checking of, 13
   information on, 13
Tongue, 18, 29-30
Torcular Herophili, 51, 53
Toxicological examination, 72-73
Tracheolaryngeal block, 30
Trauma, death from, 3, 8, 71
Treaty agreements with foreign countries, 3
Treitz, ligament of, 16, 23
Trochar marks, 69
Tuberculosis, 39
Tumor cases, 32
Tumors, 38-39, 53, 68

U
Umbilical cord, 68
Unattended patients' deaths, 8
Unclaimed body, 3
   disposition of, 3
   release for autopsy, 3
Uncles, 3
Unexpected death under care of physician, 3
Unusual deaths, 8
Ureters, 25-26, 29, 39
Urethra, 29, 39
Urinary bladder (see Bladder)
Uterus, 26, 29, 39

V
Vagina, 29, 39
Vater, ampulla, 34

Vena Cava, 20-22 fig., 29, 33
Verbal protocol, 76-78
Vertebral arteries, 51
Vertebral column, 26, 28 (see also Spinal cord)
   anterior approach to removal, 56
   block approach to removal, 55-56
   posterior approach to removal, 56
Virchow chisel, 41, 46 fig.
   evisceration, 18-28
   examination, 15-18
Viscera retention for gross organ review, 9

W
Waiting period, 3
Weighing of body, 13
Weights
   organs, 75, 115
   patient, 75
Willis, circle of, 60
Wirsung, duct of, 35
Witches' milk, 68
Witness to consent, 5
Written consents, 3, 5

X
X-rays, availability of, 75

Z
Zenker's solution, 10, 113